Revised Edition

THE COMPUTER-BASED PATIENT RECORD

An Essential Technology for Health Care

Committee on Improving the Patient Record

Division of Health Care Services

INSTITUTE OF MEDICINE

Richard S. Dick, Elaine B. Steen, and
Don E. Detmer, Editors

NATIONAL ACADEMY PRESS
Washington, D.C. 1997

NATIONAL ACADEMY PRESS · 2101 Constitution Avenue, N.W. • Washington, D.C. 20418

NOTICE: The project that is the subject of this report was approved by the Governing Board of the National Research Council, whose members are drawn from the councils of the National Academy of Sciences, the National Academy of Engineering, and the Institute of Medicine. The members of the committee responsible for the report were chosen for their special competences and with regard for appropriate balance.

The committee report and the commentaries were reviewed by groups other than the authors according to procedures approved by a Report Review Committee consisting of members of the National Academy of Sciences, the National Academy of Engineering, and the Institute of Medicine.

The Institute of Medicine was chartered in 1970 by the National Academy of Sciences to enlist distinguished members of the appropriate professions in the examination of policy matters pertaining to the health of the public. In this, the Institute acts under both the Academy's 1863 congressional charter responsibility to be an adviser to the federal government and its own initiative in identifying issues of medical care, research, and education.

See page xv for a listing of the organizations that supported the original and revised reports.

Library of Congress Cataloging-in-Publication Data

Institute of Medicine (U.S.). Committee on Improving the Patient
  Record.
    The computer-based patient record : an essential technology for
  health care / Committee on Improving the Patient Record, Division of
  Health Care Services, Institute of Medicine ; Don E. Detmer, Elaine
  B. Steen, and Richard S. Dick, editors. —Rev. ed.
      p. cm
    Includes bibliographical references and index.
    ISBN 0-309-05532-6
    1. Medical records—Data processing. I. Detmer, Don E.
  II. Steen, Elaine B. III. Dick, Richard S. IV. Title
    [DNLM: 1. Medical Records. 2. Medical Records Systems,
  Computerized—organization & administration. 3. Delivery of Health
  Care, Integrated—organization & administration. WX 173 159c 1997]
  R864.I55 1997
  651.5'04261'0285—dc21
  DNLM/DLC
  for Library of Congress   97-31030

COMMITTEE ON IMPROVING THE PATIENT RECORD IN RESPONSE TO INCREASING FUNCTIONAL REQUIREMENTS AND TECHNOLOGICAL ADVANCES

DON E. DETMER (*Chair*),* Professor of Surgery and Business Administration and Vice President for Health Sciences, University of Virginia, Charlottesville

MARION J. BALL, Associate Vice President for Information Resources, University of Maryland, Baltimore

G. OCTO BARNETT,* Professor of Medicine, Harvard Medical School, and Director, Laboratory of Computer Science, Massachusetts General Hospital, Boston

DONALD M. BERWICK, Associate Professor of Pediatrics, Harvard Medical School, Boston, Massachusetts

MORRIS F. COLLEN,* Director Emeritus and Consultant, Division of Research, Kaiser Permanente Medical Care Program, Oakland, California

NICHOLAS E. DAVIES,† Practitioner of Internal Medicine, Atlanta, Georgia

RUTH E. GARRY, Senior Manager, Group Benefits Services Division, CNA Insurance Companies, Chicago, Illinois

THOMAS Q. MORRIS, Professor of Clinical Medicine, College of Physicians and Surgeons of Columbia University, and Past President, Columbia Presbyterian Medical Center, New York, New York

JOHN A. NORRIS, Corporate Executive Vice President, Hill and Knowlton, Inc., Waltham, Massachusetts, and Lecturer in Health Law, Harvard School of Public Health, Boston, Massachusetts

EDWARD H. SHORTLIFFE,* Professor of Medicine and Computer Science; Head, Division of General Internal Medicine; and Director, Medical Information Sciences Training Program, Stanford University School of Medicine, Palo Alto, California

LIAISON MEMBERS

HENRY KRAKAUER, Director, Office of Program Assessment and Information, Health Standards and Quality Bureau, Health Care Financing Administration, Baltimore, Maryland

DONALD A. B. LINDBERG,* Director, National Library of Medicine, National Institutes of Health, Bethesda, Maryland

---

*Member, Institute of Medicine.

†Deceased, April 1991.

iii

Study Staff

Original Edition

RICHARD S. DICK, Study Director
ELAINE B. STEEN, Staff Officer
EVANSON H. JOSEPH, Project Secretary
KARL D. YORDY, Director, Division of Health Care Services
KATHLEEN N. LOHR, Deputy Director, Division of Health Care Services

Revised Edition

MARILYN J. FIELD, Deputy Director, Division of Health Care Services
KARLA SAUNDERS, Administrative Assistant

Preface—Revised Edition

The publication of a revised edition of an Institute of Medicine (IOM) report is atypical. In this case, the high, persisting demand for the original report and continued interest in computer-based patient records (CPRs) led the IOM to endorse the production of a second edition 6 years after the release of the original report. The initiation of the second report corresponded with the midway point of the target set in the recommendations of the Committee on Improving the Patient Record for achieving widespread implementation of CPRs in 10 years. Financial support from both the public and private sectors made the publication of the second edition a reality. This edition contains a new Preface, two commentaries that report on the state of CPRs today, and the full text of the original report published in 1991. The commentaries are individually authored and are not the product of a study committee, but like all IOM publications, they did undergo the standard National Academy of Sciences/National Research Council report review process. The authors of the commentaries are distinguished leaders in the field of medical informatics and are particularly well known for their work on CPRs. Drs. Paul C. Tang and W. Ed Hammond are past chairs of the Computer-based Patient Record Institute (CPRI), Dr. Jan H. van Bemmel edits the annual *Yearbook of Medical Informatics* for the International Medical Informatics Association, and Drs. Astrid M. van Ginneken and Johan van der Lei have written extensively on CPRs.

Six years has proven to be a long time in the world of health care. When the original report was released in 1991, the genetic locations of mutations that result in several major diseases were still unknown and laparoscopic surgery was just coming into widespread use. We had essentially nothing

v

to offer AIDS sufferers in the way of treatment, neither did we use umbilical cord blood for bone marrow transplantation. During these past few years comprehensive government-led health care reform reached its pinnacle, was defeated, and market-driven changes in health care financing and delivery permeated much of the country.

There have been equally significant changes in information technology. Between 1991 and 1997, there was a 8-fold increase in power and capacity of personal computers and comparable improvements in peripheral devices with the result of making powerful workstations more affordable. The dramatic strides in computer technology have been accompanied by the massive growth of the Internet, as well as of local and regional networks that link communities, schools, health care providers, and individuals to information resources around the world.

Despite this milieu of rapid change, the vision outlined in this report by the Committee on Improving the Patient Record remains remarkably on target, and the case for CPRs is stronger today than it was 6 years ago. The demand for timely, accurate health data continues to grow. The changing demographics of the population are placing more demands on the information capabilities of health care providers and systems. The increasing volume of data collected and the continued growth of medical knowledge have created a dramatic need for information technology appropriate for the task of sorting through all the information available, assessing the strength of the evidence, and bringing it to practitioners whenever they need it, particularly at the time they are making care decisions. Further, the evolution of health care delivery organizations into integrated delivery systems means that those organizations need a way of managing their services. And, of course, citizens and other purchasers need better tools for assessing the performance of health care providers as well as for managing their own health care decisions.

Looking ahead, current trends in health care delivery, management, and research will likely broaden the vision of CPRs in two areas: population-based management of health through computer-based population records and citizen-based management of health through another variant of the CPR, the computer-based personal health record. First, CPRs will play an increasingly important role in supplying data for computer-based population data bases. High-quality data are essential to the management of care for individuals; however, such data are equally critical for research, to support public health activities, and to track the performance of health care providers—both individuals and institutions. Second, as people continue to become more active consumers of health care and assume greater responsibility for managing their own health, and as information technology becomes available in more homes, individuals will increasingly use elements of the CPR and CPR-related technology to search through the health literature, communicate with their health care professionals, access data on their health care history, track the costs and value of the services they receive, diagnose acute conditions, and manage chronic conditions. The emergence of personal health information systems—customer-based personal health records—that are responsive to a variety of needs of individuals raises new opportunities for systems developers to provide complicated information in an easily understood format. Moreover, integrated delivery systems may increasingly view customer-based personal health record systems as a means of attracting new members, streamlining communication with patients, and diagnosing and monitoring patient conditions remotely and cost-effectively.

The demand for CPR systems has steadily increased since the release of the first edition of this report. CPR innovators—in the United States, Europe, and elsewhere—are proving not only that CPRs can meet users' needs, but also that there are significant benefits to be gained from their use. Recent experience has shown that access to data and information at the point of care and the ability to analyze data for management and research purposes improve the quality and reduce the costs of care. These capacities are critical for any health care provider—whether a group practice, hospital, or integrated delivery system—to function successfully. Thus, CPRs are, and will continue to be, an essential technology for health care.

Today there are several examples of quite robust hospital-based CPR systems developed by individual institutions, and commercial systems have moved toward achieving the 12 attributes of CPRs outlined in the original report. Plenty of room remains, however, to combine the depth of systems developed by institutions with easily modified, modular architecture, readily available technology, and the use of national standards. Even as CPR systems become increasingly robust, there is not, nor is there likely to be, a single CPR product that meets all the needs of a provider organization. Thus, organizations seeking CPRs face significant challenges in integrating various systems to achieve the full functionality they need. Moreover, CPR diffusion goes far beyond technology within an organization and relies at least as much on a change in culture that requires motivated, educated leadership within institutions.

Until CPR use becomes the norm for all practitioners across all provider settings as recommended in the original report, we will continue to lack the tools needed to manage the quality and costs of health care, the scientific basis for health care will continue to be undermined, and the dramatic transformation of health care so urgently required will be impeded. Thus, a major challenge facing us is to determine how to advance from where we are to where we need to be with respect to the development and diffusion of CPRs. How can we take full advantage of the lessons learned by the leaders in CPR development and reduce the problems for future CPR users?

Where should we as individuals and organizations interested in achieving the potential of CPRs devote our time and financial resources?

The two commentaries give readers an opportunity to reflect on these questions. In the first chapter of this edition, Drs. Tang and Hammond describe environmental changes that reinforce the need for CPRs, review developments in the United States since 1991, and provide insight into remaining challenges. In the second chapter, Drs. van Bemmel, van Ginneken, and van der Lei describe the state of CPRs in Europe. In so doing, they highlight areas in which efforts in the United States can benefit from European experience; for example, the entire European community has a ubiquitous privacy law whereas the United States cannot seem to accomplish this important objective. They also report that there has been more activity on CPR systems for generalists compared to the United States, where the early focus of CPR development efforts was heavily tilted toward the hospital environment. Not surprisingly, both chapters emphasize the need for collaboration to further refine CPRs.

The commentaries also provide a sense of the impact of the recommendations in the original report. Briefly, varying degrees of progress can be observed on the seven recommendations originally made in Chapter 5 of this report. First, some institutions have implemented computer systems that fulfill many of the desirable functions of a CPR as their standard record for patient care; other institutions and providers are using both paper and computer systems, but see CPRs as inevitable. Second, since its creation in 1992, CPRI has been a focal point for CPR issues and has grappled with the challenges of expanding the understanding of the pivotal role of CPRs in health care delivery and of eliminating key barriers to CPR diffusion. Toward that end, in November 1996, CPRI organized a CPR summit with other major health informatics organizations to ratify and endorse actions that will overcome barriers to effective use of information technology in health care. The summit was successful in generating a high degree of consensus for immediate action.

Third, support for CPR research and development for CPRs exists, but it has not been provided in the scope and scale necessary to enable major breakthroughs. Federal funding in the United States has been modest and inconsistent; it is typically focused on research issues and is not always directly related to the development of working CPR systems. In general, private health foundations have been distressingly slow to invest their resources in this critical area and the potential for collaboration between the public and private sectors to direct policy and to leverage resources has not been achieved.

Fourth, although work on various standards has been steady and limited progress is evident, setting standards remains an arduous process with limited financial support. Moreover, a greater focus on international standards is needed. Fifth, federal laws related to CPRs (e.g., data ownership, responsibility, and confidentiality) are still lacking. At least in the case of protection of personal health data, lively discussion and debate have prevented a consensus leading to the enactment of sound policy. On a more positive note, however, the United States Department of Health and Human Services has created a high-level data council, and its National Committee on Vital and Health Statistics is refocusing its efforts on the handling of data in part through the mandate of Public Law 104-191, the Health Insurance Portability and Accountability Act.

Sixth, no progress can be reported on the recommendation that the costs of developing and implementing CPRs should be shared among those who benefit from them. The cost of capitalizing CPR systems remains a significant hurdle for individual institutions, and it is a serious policy issue that must be addressed. Finally, anecdotal evidence indicates that there are better educational opportunities for health care professionals to acquire the skills necessary to develop and use CPRs. There is, however, an equally important need to educate administrators and other people involved in allocating resources to and selecting CPR systems about both the benefits and complexities of CPR systems.

An important issue emerges after reviewing the limited impact of the committee's seven recommendations over the past 6 years. What else needs to be done to advance CPRs? What would help to jumpstart this process and expedite progress toward the committee's original goal of widespread implementation of CPRs by 2001? Again, the commentaries shed light on these questions. The original report called for federal support of CPRI, public and private support of research and development, federal laws related to CPRs, and collaboration among various public and private groups to explore CPR reimbursement mechanisms.

As Drs. Tang and Hammond report, individual federal agencies have played a role over the past few years, but a coordinated, comprehensive, funded policy has not emerged. In contrast, Drs. van Bemmel, van Ginneken, and van der Lei report on several specific ways in which the European Union is supporting CPR development. Thus, in the United States, we need to establish the appropriate role of government, particularly the federal government, in advancing the development and implementation of CPRs.

A coordinated national program for CPR advancement in the United States could be based on the seven recommendations presented in the original report. Such a program would build on existing private-sector efforts and strengthen them by bringing both policy and funding leverage that the private sector cannot provide alone. As was emphasized in the original report, the federal government should not take exclusive control of CPR development and implementation; the private sector's perspectives are vital to a sound approach to CPR development.

Several of the remaining critical impediments to CPR development outlined in the commentary by Drs. Tang and Hammond are not just intractable, but virtually impossible to overcome, if pursued by the private sector alone. Moreover, crucial incremental efforts are more likely to succeed in the context of a comprehensive national program. There is every reason to push for increased government involvement without delay so that quality, cost, and access to modern, evidence-based health care can be achieved. The original 10-year target remains within reach, but only if a national effort is undertaken immediately.

Significant challenges abound: building the requisite infrastructure, optimizing the available technology (including integrating various systems), ensuring the availability of enough people with the right skills, addressing organizational culture and change issues, and confronting financing and policy issues. Clearly, this most essential of all elements of modern health care—a robust CPR—has a growing body of advocates. The challenge is to coalesce these parties into a public-private partnership dedicated to creating through the information infrastructure a better health care system for all Americans. As the Preface to the first edition concluded,

> Success will require cooperation and coordination, and perhaps some sacrifice and compromise as well, but we are fully convinced that the outcomes will be well worth such an effort. What we believe will emerge will be a more caring, more scientific, and no less important, more cost-effective health care system. (*Pp. vi-vii*)

We hope that this report will continue to be a catalyst to encourage people to take advantage of the opportunity at hand. We must move from debate and discussion about the remaining impediments to education, investment, and most important, to action by both the private and public sectors to realize the potential of the CPR as an—perhaps the—essential technology for health care.

Don E. Detmer, M.D., and Elaine B. Steen, M.A.

Preface—Original Edition

Health care professionals and policymakers seeking to ensure greater value in health care services face many boundary conditions that are fixed and a host of problems that are not. Today, the opportunity to affect one of those boundary conditions—the information management capabilities in health care—is within our grasp. This report advocates the prompt development and implementation of computer-based patient records (CPRs). Put simply, this Institute of Medicine committee believes that CPRs and CPR systems have a unique potential to improve the care of both individual patients and populations and, concurrently, to reduce waste through continuous quality improvement.

We are not suggesting a simple automation of the current patient record. Rather, we envision the next generation of CPRs and CPR systems as essential to the full maturation of the scientific basis of health care. The report outlines the basic components of future CPRs and a strategic plan for achieving widespread CPR implementation. Further, it identifies the key organizations that will need to play major roles if the plan is to succeed.

The vision of the patient record of the future that emerged from the committee's deliberations seems uniquely appropriate for a nation that values pluralism and privacy and has a mobile population with growing levels of chronic illness. CPRs are a key infrastructural requirement to support the information management needs of physicians, other health professionals, and a variety of other legitimate users of aggregated patient information. It is this vision, as much as any other message, that the committee hopes will engage the reader. We believe that if enough individuals become embued with this sense of the possible, the reality will emerge.

Our report is intended for a very broad audience. We see it as especially pertinent for physicians and other health care practitioners; health care managers; medical record professionals; health services researchers; medical informatics researchers; computer vendors; third-party payers; the legal community; federal, state, and local health care agencies; state legislators; members of the federal legislative and executive branches of government; and, finally, interested citizens. All these parties, we believe, have much to gain from the success of CPRs and CPR systems.

Happily, this report complements and is complemented by several other recent activities that convinced us, as we proceeded with our work, that the time was ripe for a major CPR initiative. The Office of Science and Data Development of the Agency for Health Care Policy and Research (AHCPR) is leading efforts to improve the quality and quantity of data available for health services research—particularly effectiveness, appropriateness, and outcomes research. In addition, the AHCPR Forum on Quality and Effectiveness in Health Care, the American Medical Association, and other professional organizations are playing a major national role in the development of clinical practice guidelines. The CPR will be a boon to both these endeavors.

The activities of several other groups also lend support to the move toward widespread implementation of computer-based records. The General Accounting Office recently released a forward-looking report on the potential benefits of patient record automation. Several Institute of Medicine reports published over the last two years cite the need for improved patient data collection to support quality assurance, utilization management, and effectiveness research. The National Science Foundation recently issued a report on the benefits of a national system for very high speed data communication, including health data. Finally, the National Research Council's recently released report on safe computing in the information age outlines problems and opportunities in computer security.

Given this apparent climate of opportunity for CPR development and implementation, the committee came to the end of its work eager to disseminate its message regarding the feasibility and potential of CPRs and CPR systems. The natural ebullience common to the conclusion of a study was tempered, however, by the untimely death of committee member Nicholas E. Davies. Dr. Davies saw more clearly than many of us what needed to be done to implement the vision of fully developed patient records and had committed his considerable personal energies to achieving our collective goals for CPRs and CPR systems. For this reason we feel it appropriate to dedicate this report to him and to his belief in our vision.

If this project is to succeed, we must soon see organizational efforts that adopt and implement, or refine and implement, our recommendations. Success will require cooperation and coordination, and perhaps some sacrifice and compromise as well, but we are fully convinced that the outcomes will be well worth such an effort. What we believe will emerge will be a more caring, more scientific, and, no less important, more cost-effective health care system. We hope that this report will be a catalyst to encourage you to join with us to address the opportunity at hand.

Finally, on a personal note, the enthusiasm, involvement, and support of the many individuals and institutions acknowledged elsewhere in this report were deeply appreciated.

Don E. Detmer, M.D.
Chair

Acknowledgments—Revised Edition

This revised report was an unusual effort stimulated by both the widespread interest in the original committee report and the rapid pace of developments since the publication of that report. In addition to the authors of the two commentaries, the editors want to acknowledge the contributions of Octo Barnett, M.D., Harvard University, who substantially strengthened the commentaries through his rigorous review. At the Institute of Medicine, Marilyn J. Field, Ph.D., Deputy Director of the Division of Health Care Services, offered to steer the revised report through the various stages of fundraising, editing, report review, and publication. Karla Saunders worked with drafts of the national and international commentaries to prepare them for review and for publication. Claudia Carl, Mike Edington, and Mona Brinegar provided additional assistance at various stages in the process. Margret Amatyakul, Executive Director of the Computer-based Patient Record Institute, was instrumental in helping to raise funds and otherwise support this revised edition.

Support for this revised edition was provided by the National Library of Medicine and the Centers for Disease Control and Prevention through the Computer-based Patient Record Institute. Additional support was provided by the Joint Commission on Accreditation of Healthcare Organizations, Oceania, Inc., American Board of Family Practice, Inc., MedicaLogic, Inc., 3M, Association of Operating Room Nurses, Inc., Adventist Health System Sunbelt Health Care Corporation, Computer-based Patient Record Institute, Inc., American Health Information Management Association, Ernst & Young LLP, and Hewlett-Packard.

Support for the committee report (original edition) was provided by the

American Medical Record Association, Baxter Healthcare Corporation, Booz-Allen and Hamilton, E. I. du Pont de Nemours and Company, Gerber Alley and Company, the John A. Hartford Foundation, Hewlett-Packard Company, IBM Corporation, Kaiser Foundation Hospitals, and Science Applications International Corporation. In addition, the Health Care Financing Administration (Contract No. 500-90-0041), the Department of Veterans Affairs (Contract No. 101-C90014), and the Health Resources and Services Administration provided financial support. Finally, the Agency for Health Care Policy and Research (Contract No. 282-90-0018) provided funds for a workshop that contributed to the deliberations of the study committee; the former National Center for Health Services Research provided funds for planning efforts before the study began (Grant No. 5909 HS055 2602).

Acknowledgments—Original Edition

The committee would like to express its appreciation for the contributions of many individuals and organizations to this project. In addition to the subcommittee members listed in Appendix A, more than 200 individuals representing organizations throughout the health care sector attended subcommittee meetings or submitted written information, providing the committee with a broad base of information from which to draw. Several subcommittee members led work groups or prepared papers and presentations. Subcommittee chairs and assistant chairs in particular devoted significant amounts of time preparing for their meetings and writing reports of subcommittee findings for use by the full study committee.

Several individuals prepared background papers that were most helpful to the study committee and staff. In addition to Adele Waller (whose paper appears in this volume), the committee acknowledges the contributions of Paul Tang, Donald Lindberg and Betsy Humphreys, Margret Amatayakul and Mary Joan Wogan, John Silva, and Orley Lindgren and Don Harper Mills. The committee also expresses its gratitude to the participants of a workshop on overcoming barriers to patient record development who provided the committee with a sounding board for its ideas about an organizational framework to accelerate such development.

This study would not have been possible without financial support from many entities. Within the private sector, we acknowledge generous support from the American Medical Record Association, Baxter Healthcare Corporation, Booz-Allen and Hamilton, E. I. du Pont de Nemours and Company, Gerber Alley and Company, the John A. Hartford Foundation, Hewlett-Packard Company, IBM Corporation, Kaiser Foundation Hospitals, and Science Applications International Corporation. Within the public sector, the Department of Veterans Affairs, the Health Care Financing Administration, and the Health Resources and Services Administration provided important funding for the study. The Agency for Health Care Policy and Research (AHCPR) sponsored a workshop on overcoming barriers to patient record development that provided valuable information for the committee's deliberations. Preliminary staff work on the study was supported in part by the Institute of Medicine Council on Health Care Technology, which received financial support from AHCPR's predecessor, the National Center for Health Services Research and Health Care Technology Assessment.

We are indebted to several Institute of Medicine staff members. Enriqueta Bond and Richard Rettig oversaw the initiation of the project. Maria Elena Lara and Ethan Halm provided staff support, and Clifford Goodman (now with the Swedish Council on Technology Assessment in Health Care) provided guidance in the early stages of the study. Karl Yordy, and particularly Kathleen Lohr, helped steer the study through its later phases. Elaine Steen and Richard Dick provided staff support throughout the study and were responsible for preparing this report on behalf of the committee.

All studies rely on the efforts of administrative and financial staff for day-to-day operations. The committee appreciates the contributions of Holly Dawkins, Suzanna Gilbert, Evanson Joseph, Theresa Nally, Delores Sutton, and H. Donald Tiller in project administration and Cynthia Abel, Lisa Chimento, and Nina Spruill in financial administration. Finally, we thank Leah Mazade for her editorial comments on this report.

Contents

THE
COMPUTER-BASED
PATIENT RECORD

Commentary

A Progress Report on Computer-Based Patient Records in the United States

Paul C. Tang and W. Ed Hammond

Much has changed since the release of the first edition of *The Computer-Based Patient Record: An Essential Technology for Health Care.* The current environment in which health care is practiced and the information technology available to its practitioners are significantly different from that which existed when the study was completed in 1991. Changes in the health care environment produced fundamental shifts in the delivery of health care, favoring outpatient care over inpatient care, primary care over specialty care, and guidelines-driven care over autonomous decisionmaking. Technological advances have overcome some barriers to computer-based patient records (CPRs) (e.g., World Wide Web, applications that operate across distances on many different computers) and heightened the visibility of others (e.g., confidentiality policies and legislation). In this commentary, we describe some of the environmental and technological changes that have occurred since publication of the first edition and highlight the challenges that remain to be adressed. Probably the most significant nontechnological change that occurred since 1991 was the change in the health care practice environment. We begin by addressing the new environment.

THE CHANGING HEALTH CARE LANDSCAPE: REINFORCING THE NEED FOR CPRS

As health care costs in the United States approached $1 trillion in the early 1990s, businesses, consumers, and payers began to call for mechanisms to manage the escalating costs (IOM, 1993). This issue was so much at the forefront of U.S. business and political priorities, that the 1992 presidential election was dominated by discussions of health care costs and debate on effective ways to control them.

Although efforts at full-scale health care reform led by the federal government gained momentum, peaked, and then disintegrated, market-driven changes in health care delivery were already under way and steadily moving forward. Managed care plans continue to gain increasing shares of the market (Hoechst Marion Rousell, Inc., 1995). The need to examine and manage the health needs of a population has dramatically increased the demand for information systems that capture clinical data. The health care information systems industry has shifted its attention from financial systems to clinical systems, particularly CPR systems. Two core tenets of managed care that impact the demand for CPR systems have been the central role of primary care and the emergence of integrated delivery systems.

The Evolving Role of Primary Care

Managed care has redefined the primary care provider as the principal provider of care and, in many instances, a gatekeeper for access to certain diagnostic tests and specialty care. To efficiently carry out these roles, the clinician needs ready access to both clinical and administrative data. At the same time, guidelines are being promoted to reduce the variances among clinical practices. When guidelines are integrated into a CPR system, they can streamline the steps necessary to adhere to them and simultaneously document that compliance. CPR systems that integrate clinical guidelines in the order-entry process have the best acceptance among providers (Sittig and Stead, 1994; Sullivan and Mitchell, 1995; CPRI, 1996c, 1997). However, despite the abundance of guidelines, few can be implemented in a computer as written (Tierney et al., 1995). Software tools are needed to help author guidelines that are internally consistent, include precise definitions of eligibility criteria, and accommodate a variety of patient conditions.

One of the major goals of managed care is to provide more of the care outside of the hospital. However, the inpatient and the outpatient settings differ substantially. There are differences in the temporal nature of information, the responsibilities of each member of the health care team, the need for a communications infrastructure to facilitate coordination of care, and other logistical concerns which impact the detailed design of information systems. Consequently, vendors of information system products for hospitals find that there is a steep learning curve to understanding the information needs of physicians in the ambulatory care setting. Deliberate analysis of the information needs and work flow requirements in ambulatory care will help system developers design information systems that increase the efficiency and effectiveness of clinical practice throughout the continuum.

The Integrated Delivery System

Another fundamental concept that heightens the need for CPR systems is that of an integrated delivery system (IDS). An IDS is composed of health care providers, service providers, and facilities organized to provide a continuum of health care services to a defined population. These systems of health care were created in response to payers' desire to contract with single entities that provide comprehensive health care services for their clients. To manage the delivery of care in an IDS, a health system must have efficient and accurate ways of capturing, managing, and analyzing clinical data collected at all the different sites where care is provided.

In addition, payers and regulators are requesting "report cards" on quality, outcomes, and costs of care provided by the integrated delivery system. For example, the National Committee for Quality Assurance (NCQA) developed the Health Plan Employer Data and Information Set (HEDIS) as a standard report card to help employers evaluate different health plans. Initially focused more on administrative data, the evolving HEDIS criteria are increasingly targeting clinical processes and outcomes. Gathering the data to prepare these reports can be immensely time-consuming and costly when they are manually abstracted from paper records, but with a CPR, reporting on aggregate data can be a byproduct of capturing data electronically.

NCQA advised health plans to "move to fully implement the information framework, including the automated patient record" in order to meet the clinical reporting requirements of forthcoming regulations (NCQA, 1997). As outcomes reporting requirements become more sophisticated and deal with complex, multifaceted diseases, it will be essential to have electronic access to the record and tools to efficiently analyze practice patterns and patient outcomes. NCQA will develop HEDIS measures that assume health plans and provider organizations use CPRs by 2002.

In short, since the release of the first edition, the demand for clinical data has become a business imperative. The organizational complexities of these large, diverse, and geographically dispersed health systems add new challenges—and new opportunities—for developers and implementers of CPR systems.

Technological Advances

Computer processing power doubles in performance and halves in cost about every 2 years. These past 6 years have been no exception. Although it is not our intent to review all the developments in information technology (because technology has not been the critical impediment to adoption of CPR systems), three striking technological shifts have occurred that favorably impact the foundation for CPR systems. We briefly describe these developments below.

The Internet and the World Wide Web: Widespread Connectivity

Perhaps the single biggest technological change since the first edition of the report is the rising importance of the Internet. Although the Internet dates back to 1969 when the first node of ARPANET was installed at the University of California at Los Angeles, several changes have coalesced to bring together a paradigm shift that now touches all segments of society. The World Wide Web (WWW) has transformed a research network into the fabric of a new information age. Internet service providers have made access convenient and reasonably inexpensive. As much as 50 percent of the U.S. population will have access to the Internet by early in the next century (National Research Council, 1996). It is precisely this kind of ubiquitous connectivity that enables IDS organizations to share data throughout their geographically dispersed clinical delivery sites, and even to reach the consumer or patient at home. To the extent that health care becomes dependent on access to computer networks, however, policymakers need to pay special attention to the needs of the medically underserved population to ensure that lack of network access does not further impede their access to care.

Connectivity is not the only requirement for transmitting patient data to remote sites. Confidentiality and security safeguards need to be developed and enforced. Fortunately, the requirements of business to protect electronic commerce over the Internet will drive technical solutions and policy standards, which health care applications can leverage. Technology dedicated solely to health care applications risk being orphaned due to the lack of a mass market. The market drive of consumerism must pave the information infrastructure for health care applications

World Wide Web Browsers: A Universal View on the Internet

Probably the most important tool that led to the domestication of the Internet was the development of software that made it easy to connect to, search, browse, and download information from anywhere on the network as if it were located on the user's personal computer. Commonly called browser software (e.g., Netscape Navigator™, Microsoft Internet Explorer™), these programs give a graphical, intuitive, and common interface to functions that locate and interact with remote data on the Internet without the user having any technical knowledge of how it is done. Browser user interfaces have become so commonplace that they are being adopted as the interface to desktop computers.

Another fundamental breakthrough associated with WWW browsers is that the software runs on almost any computer (Cimino, 1995). One of the critical problems that had been plaguing computer users since the invention of electronic computing has been the general inability of programs written for one machine to run on another machine or to use data generated by another program. Efficient and cost-effective use of computers suffered due to the incompatibilities caused by a lack of standards. The WWW defined standards for document formats (hypertext markup language, HTML) and transfer protocols (hypertext transfer protocol, HTTP). Compliance with these standards permitted independent developers to write programs for heterogeneous computers and operating systems, yet have them all seamlessly access information on the WWW.

The success of the WWW demonstrates the market-expanding potential of adopted standards. It also demonstrates the remarkable leverage provided through natural entrepreneurial forces complying with industry standards. The benefits to the consumer, including clinicians, are tremendous.

The Intranet

A variant, but powerful spin-off, of the Internet is the Intranet, a controlled-access version of the Internet. Like the Internet, Intranets use industry-standard document formats, data exchange protocols, and browsers. The prolific development of new tools and products for the Internet can be directly applied to Intranets. An estimated 80 percent of the Internet products are purchased for use on an Intranet. The Intranet, however, typically has better bandwidth, security, and administration because it is controlled and operated by the private enterprise. These advantages are particularly important for health care applications, and most health care organizations are exploring the use of Intranets as a component of their information strategy.

Network-Centric Computing

Industry is at the cusp of another major change—network-centric computing. The predominant paradigm for computing today uses personal computers (PCs) to perform most of the computational work using software that resides on local disks. The hardware, software, and support costs for this type of operation require large budgets and staffs.

Network-centric computers are diskless computers that attach to a network and load software stored on a server computer. The capability to manage hardware and software more centrally reduces the acquisition and operating costs for the enterprise. Although this new architecture has not been used extensively in production, it has the potential to revamp distributed computing.

Having noted the significant changes in the health care environment and advances in information technology, we next discuss the current state of the CPR.

THE CURRENT STATE OF CPRs

As discussed in Chapter 4 of the report, the development and diffusion of a new technology are separable but interrelated events. In discussing the state of CPR development and implementation in the United States today, it would be desirable to examine two questions. First, to what extent have CPRs, as defined by the study committee, been developed? Second, to what extent have the available CPRs been adopted? Unfortunately, a comprehensive review of the industry does not exist, and it would soon be out of date if it did. Alternatively, one could rephrase the questions from the perspectives of providers and vendors. From the perspective of system purchasers, do the CPR systems that are available in the market meet the needs of health care institutions? And from the perspective of vendors, is the market ready to buy CPR systems? Although in neither case is the answer a resounding "yes," promising signs can be reported.

The CPR Market

One must be careful when describing a "CPR market" not to tether the concept to a single, static idea whose incarnation can be purchased "off-the-shelf." In some sense, it is precisely the static nature of the paper-based record that has been such a great burden to the practice of medicine. Instead, a CPR system is a constantly evolving concept whose value and function is expected to grow with the constantly changing demands of the health care environment and the improving technology upon which the system is built. The level of CPR development activity has definitely increased significantly since 1991. The number of commercial systems addressing various attributes of CPRs has increased and most major health care information technology vendors now offer CPR-related products. However, comprehensive information system products that seamlessly integrate data and coordinate processes across the entire continuum of health care services do not exist. Most health care information system vendors, whether their products were formerly based in the inpatient or the outpatient side, are working to extend their products to cover the needs of integrated delivery systems. Developers generally start from the data end of the system and work toward the human side where the clinician interacts directly with the system. Hence, one way to trace the evolving functionality is to look at the transformation of data into information that clinicians use to make decisions. Although the path is not necessarily sequential, five hallmarks of this transformation are enumerated below:

1. Integrated view of patient data,
2. Access to knowledge resources,
3. Physician order entry and clinician data entry,
4. Integrated communications support, and
5. Clinical decision support.

Integrated View of Patient Data

This is one of the earliest benefits of CPRs—improving access to all patient data whenever and wherever clinical decisions are made independent of where the data was originally acquired. Observational studies of clinicians' information needs provide details on the kinds of information physicians require to make decisions regarding the care of their patients (Tang et al., 1994). Up to 81 percent of the time, physicians could not find all the available patient information desired to make patient care decisions during an outpatient encounter. Limited by a format that has not substantively changed in close to a century, the paper record is ill-suited to the information demands of modern clinical practice. Most CPR system vendors offer products that combine data from various sources and present an integrated view to clinicians.

Access to Knowledge Resources

Providers often need other information in addition to patient data and their own personal knowledge (Covell et al., 1985). The guidelines, rules, and regulations in the managed care environment have intensified this need to access medical and administrative knowledge at the time decisions are made. CPR systems sometimes provide methods for organizations to incorporate access to local knowledge resources, but generally, this knowledge access is passive. That is, the user searches for the needed information electronically but has to abstract the pertinent content and enter any relevant orders manually into the clinical system. Ideally, access to knowledge resources should be integrated with clinical decision support in ways that directly influence physicians' ordering behavior, as described below.

Physician Order Entry and Clinician Data Entry

Physician orders initiate clinical interventions. Proactively influencing physicians' orders is the most efficient way to influence patient outcomes (McDonald, 1976, 1984). Systems that physicians use routinely to enter orders, whether in the inpatient setting or outpatient setting, can produce significant effects on quality and costs of care (Barnett, 1984; Tierney et al., 1987, 1990, 1993; Sittig and Stead, 1994). In addition, when clinical data are entered and maintained by the clinicians responsible for care, the accuracy and quality of data are high. Very few commercial systems, however, are used by physicians to write all their orders. Human-computer interface issues and perceived benefit substantially affect the success of this function. Some of the reasons are discussed later under remaining barriers.

Integrated Communications Support

With an increasing emphasis on outpatient care, coordinating the activities of health care professionals from multiple organizations at different sites, including the home, becomes more important. No longer confined to an acute care facility where proximity between the health care team members and the patient was the rule, the patient and care team in the outpatient setting meet more by appointment than by clinical demand. Relying on paper-based mail is inefficient and fallible. Clinicians need integrated communications support for effective functioning of the multidisciplinary outpatient health care team (Tang et al., 1996). A communications infrastructure that is linked to the shared patient record facilitates overall coordination of care and timely response to changing patient conditions.

Clinical Decision Support

Few, if any, commercial systems provide a high level of proactive decision support. Drug interaction checking and simple abnormal laboratory-test result alerts are available, but the richness of applying a broad range of knowledge to influence physicians' orders is still under development (Johnson, 1994).

Only when both patient data and clinical knowledge reside in the system in machine-understandable format can the system provide additional support to the clinician making decisions. For example, encoded medical knowledge about the meaning and significance of changing laboratory-test results would allow a system to provide alerts, an active function, in addition to the passive data retrieval function. Similarly, if the system could match the patient context with relevant clinical guidelines, it could present ordering options consistent with the appropriate guidelines. The clinician is responsible for the definitive decision, but the system can actively provide options and explanations that improve the clinician's efficiency and compliance with accepted guidelines of practice.

In summary, since the first edition, there has been a significant increase in development efforts on CPR systems. We remain optimistic that the remaining years of the decade-long challenge will deliver on the promises of computer-supported decisionmaking.

At the Fork

In 1991, the Committee on Improving the Patient Record reported that the most advanced CPR systems were found in several academic medical centers or teaching hospitals affiliated with universities as well as in the Department of Veterans Affairs and the Department of Defense. Not surprisingly, today the most advanced CPR systems implemented in the United States can be found in the same places. Of the seven institutions that have been recognized as part of the Computer-based Patient Record Institute Davies CPR Recognition Program (described below), four are academic medical centers and one is the Department of Veterans Affairs. One of the distinguishing factors of institutions that have been recognized as having advanced CPRs is the clear organizational leadership and commitment to CPR system implementation that helped make their efforts successful (CPRI, 1995c, 1996c, 1997).

A comic saying attributed to Yogi Berra states: "When you come to the fork in the road, take it." In contrast to the early CPR system adopters, most health care institutions are standing at the fork, trying to decide whether or not to begin implementing a CPR system. Those who have made the decision to invest in a CPR system are grappling with the complicated issue of how to do so. Many organizations implement the CPR system in some, but not all areas. Others implement a partial system and depend on a combination of paper and electronic documentation. All adopters of CPR systems must address how to integrate the components of the CPR and how to integrate the CPR with other institutional information systems. The challenge of implementing such an expansive, robust system is daunting, but the option of continuing to manage the clinical and administrative data of an IDS on paper is increasingly becoming a nonviable alternative.

Recent Activity to Advance CPRs in the United States

Against the backdrop of technical and nontechnical changes, interest in and incentives to develop CPR systems have increased.

The National Library of Medicine (NLM) has been at the forefront in stimulating research on the effective use of CPR systems and networked access to shared data (Lindberg, 1995). NLM conducts intramural research that is directly applicable to technological and infrastructural needs of CPR system development and effectively uses its extramural research grants and contracts to apply the results of academic research to health care. Through its High-Performance Computing and Communications contracts, NLM has been a leader in facilitating the use of information technology by health care professionals of rural, urban, community, and statewide networks around the country. NLM's extensive work on the Unified Medical Language System (UMLS) has been a major contribution in the medical terminology arena. NLM and the Agency for Health Care Policy Research (AHCPR) are sponsoring a large-scale vocabulary test to assess the "extent to which a combination of existing health-related classifications and vocabularies covers vocabulary needed in information systems supporting health care, public health, and health services research" (Humphreys et al., 1996). NLM is further extending the reach of shared computer-based patient data and systems through its telemedicine program.

Due to AHCPR's role in developing scientifically based clinical guidelines, it has long recognized the importance of standard data definitions and capturing clinical data in structured form. AHCPR has also played an active role in facilitating standards development. Widespread use of CPR systems would not only facilitate the collection of aggregate data in support of guidelines development, but also make effective the dissemination and use of clinical guidelines in clinical practice.

In addition to the efforts undertaken by NLM and AHCPR, other federal agencies, including the Department of Defense, and the National Institute of Standards and Testing have internal and extramural activities in CPR systems. However, a cohesive federal policy to speed the development of a health information infrastructure and the diffusion of CPRs has not emerged in the United States (Shortliffe et al., 1996).

One focal point for accelerating the development of the infrastructure for CPR systems (e.g., confidentiality policies, standards, evaluation criteria) in the private sector has been the Computer-based Patient Records Institute (CPRI). CPRI was formed in response to the recommendation of the Institute of Medicine (IOM) study committee to promote and facilitate the development, implementation, and dissemination of the CPR. Led by many of the initial supporters of the IOM committee, CPRI was incorporated in January 1992, as an association of organizations representing the various stakeholders in health care. In its first year, 22 organizations became members of CPRI. Over the subsequent years, the organization has grown to more than 70 members. CPRI was charged by the IOM committee with the following objectives:

1. Support the effective, efficient use of computer-based patient records.
2. Educate change agents and stakeholders about the value of CPRs in improving patient care.
3. Foster the CPR as the primary vehicle for collecting patient data.
4. Promote the development and use of standards for CPR security and data content, structures, and vocabulary.

Despite efforts in the public and private sectors, however, significant barriers impede the development and use of CPR systems in the United States. Many of the remaining critical barriers to CPR system development and routine use concern problems that are most effectively dealt with by cooperative, focused activity. We describe some of these barriers below.

Remaining Barriers or Challenges

Technology has continued to move forward at a rapid pace. By comparison, the human and organizational sides of the challenges have remained relatively stagnant. In 1991, the committee stated that informational, organizational, and behavioral barriers must be addressed to advance CPR systems, and that these barriers overshadowed the technical barriers. Below, we elaborate on some of the critical barriers to CPR development and diffusion.

Definition of the CPR

Although work on a common definition of a CPR and CPR system is under way by various groups, a universal understanding of the concepts embodied in a

CPR does not exist. Without a clear understanding, users have a difficult time selecting systems that will meet their needs and vendors have difficulty supplying such systems. CPRI described a CPR as "electronically stored information about an individual's lifetime health status and health care." It replaces the paper medical record as the primary record of care, meeting all clinical, legal, and administrative requirements. A CPR system provides reminders and alerts, linkages with knowledge sources for decision support, and data for outcomes research and improved management of health care delivery. It is worth repeating a point made earlier that a CPR system is an evolving concept that responds to the dynamic nature of the health care environment and takes advantage of technological advances.

Beyond the first set of definitions, however, few details have been worked out and agreed upon. For example, there is no common data model for the CPR, no common set of data elements, no common vocabulary, and no common set of scenarios that are supported. These requirements are fundamental if developers are to create a person-centered CPR that links care across different sites, specialties, and circumstances.

Many systems still follow the traditional organization and characteristics of the paper-based system and have simply automated that system. Narrative documentation, for example, is far more prevalent than structured text. Even though most new CPRs support a multimedia record, new data forms have not been smoothly integrated into the record, and little has been done to evaluate their true worth. Finally, the concept of incorporating patient-derived information (e.g., health status) as part of the patient record has not been implemented to any significant degree.

Meeting User Needs

In order for clinicians to rely on data in the system, they must be the direct users of the system. The emphasis on clinical data is a fundamental change from the previous era of hospital information systems, where clerks were the main users because the primary motivation was to capture charges and generate bills.

Analysis of the common questions concerning patient information that physicians ask (e.g., what evidence supports the diagnosis, has a patient ever had a specific test, and has there been any follow-up because of a particular laboratory test result?) provides insight into the difficulties clinicians have had finding the answers in the paper-based chart. Although current computer-based tools installed in health care institutions can typically help clinicians retrieve laboratory test results, they are not designed to answer many of the common questions clinicians ask about patient data. CPR system developers will need to address these needs to satisfy the new clinician users. The maker of the Swiss Army Knife describes the key to inventions as follows: "Make it useful. Very useful. Conveniently useful. . . . " Likewise, key to gaining clinician user acceptance is providing efficient tools that help clinicians retrieve and understand data relevant to their decision-making tasks.

Clinicians also need answers to many questions regarding medical knowledge (Covell et al., 1985). Diagnostic decision support tools are available as stand-alone microcomputer programs (e.g., QMR, Illiad, DXplain) or are available over the Internet (e.g., DXplain; Miller et al., 1986; Barnett et al., 1987; Feldman and Barnett, 1991; Berner et al., 1996). However, their greatest use would occur when proven diagnostic decision support tools are integrated with CPR systems.

Among the more challenging issues confronting CPR system developers is the issue of effective user-computer interfaces. Physicians must be the users of the system, performing data entry (e.g., orders, progress notes) as well as information retrieval, if they are to realize the benefits of interactive, on-line decision support. Progress must be made in understanding the "cognitive processes involved in human-computer interactions in order to design interfaces that are more intuitive and more acceptable" (Tang and Patel, 1994). Cognitive issues are also relevant to designing the presentation of clinical information in ways that facilitate rapid assimilation and analysis. Ultimately, good solutions to the human-computer interface will require changes not only in how the system looks but also in how humans interact with the system. What information the provider needs and what tasks the provider is performing will influence what is presented as well as how it is presented. Templates that reflect providers' work flows will aid them in using the system efficiently. Defaults that represent common, desired selections, for example, not only improve efficiency but also help increase compliance with practice-defined guidelines (CPRI, 1996c, 1997).

Although user acceptance was a major barrier in the past, more and more users are demanding that organizations implement computer-based means for accessing and managing patient data. This is not to say that the cultural and organizational challenges associated with major change are not substantial barriers to overcome, but the users' awareness of the potential benefits will become an increasing catalyst for change.

The change in users and uses has a dramatic impact on the applications desired and the kinds of user interfaces required. The industry must now focus on a completely different set of users and must define and address their information needs. Proactive and informed user participation will be necessary for implementations to succeed. The attention to clinical data and clinical users described in this report is even more important today than it was 6 years ago.

Standards

Rather than existing as a monolithic system, contemporary health care information systems are made up of multiple-component systems manufactured by multiple vendors, owned by multiple entities. To share data, which is required in an IDS, industry-adopted standards must be defined for interfaces between components (AMIA, 1994; Hammond, 1994).

Health systems must have a unique health identifier (UHI) to accurately and reliably link all the data on a single individual. Until last year, striving for a national UHI had been an elusive goal. Public Law 104-191 (The Insurance Portability and Accountability Act of 1996) calls for the secretary of Health and Human Services "to adopt standards for unique health identifiers, confidentiality policies, and terminology." To build support for addressing these pivotal issues, in November 1996, CPRI convened a national Summit of over 80 senior executives representing health care providers, health systems, government agencies, information systems vendors, businesses, regulators, and quality assurance professionals. The organizations participating in the Summit developed consensus recommendations regarding a unique health identifier, confidentiality legislation and policies, and standard health terminology. CPRI was charged with follow-up actions to work with government agencies and industry groups to implement the recommendations.

The need for standards governing the content, vocabulary, and format of data remains a high priority. So far, most of the progress has been made in the development of messaging standards. Standards for data exchange have continued to be expanded and are increasingly being adopted by provider organizations and vendors. Standards now exist for exchanging clinical data (Health Level Seven [HL-7], 1994), images (ACR/NEMA), clinical observations (ASTM Committee E-31), bedside instrument data (IEEE, 1995), prescription data (NCPDP, 1992), and administrative data associated with claims (Accredited Standards Committee X12N). It is important to note, however, that even with standards that define message formats, implementation of messaging standards may differ among vendors. The next step is to call on industry to provide standard implementations for messaging standards such as HL-7. That would be a major step toward "plug-and-play" capability.

Although there has been progress in developing individual coding standards for data elements, none has emerged as a comprehensive standard. More than 150 different coding sets defining terms for use with the medical record have been created. Among these coding sets are ICD9-CM, ICD10, SNOMED III, CPT, NANDA, Read Classification, LOINC, and MEDRA, to name a few. Not only findings, but also results of laboratory tests must have standard terms (e.g., results of a Pap smear or mammogram). Additional coding sets are being defined by specialty groups that recognize the need for a common vocabulary. The NLM has expanded its UMLS to map many of these coding sets into a common set. Names for every element that must be exchanged among systems should be standardized. For the CPR, a clinically rich vocabulary that accurately describes patient problems and findings is mandatory. In addition, physicians must feel comfortable with the standard vocabulary if they are to use it for entering data. CPRI has published an evaluation of existing comprehensive codes (Chute et al., 1996).

In addition to standards for patient data, medical knowledge must be encoded in CPR systems with decision support capability. The Arden syntax has been used to exchange medical knowledge encoded as simple rules (Hripcsak et al., 1990). Further work must be undertaken to represent medical knowledge in standard, transferable form.

Leadership at the federal level is required to ensure that standards necessary to preserve and enhance health care in the United States are developed. Until standards exist for uniquely identifying individuals and coding and exchanging health data, the value from capturing and aggregating data will go unrealized and each organization will be its own pioneer.

Legal and Social Issues

Security, privacy, and confidentiality concerns have become major barriers to widespread implementation of CPR systems and sharing data. There is, as yet, no agreement on what must be done to establish the balance between appropriate use of health care data and the individual patient's rights to privacy (Detmer and Steen, 1996). The issue of who owns the data in a CPR is still being debated. Of equal importance to preserving patient privacy and confidentiality is the necessity of preserving institutional privacy. No institution will be willing to share data if those data can be used to provide a business advantage for a competitor. Again, the human factors outweigh the technical solutions in dealing with this issue (Barrows and Clayton, 1996).

Privacy and confidentiality are concepts that involve people, policies, and legislation. Information security technology plays an enabling and facilitating role by helping organizations prevent unauthorized access to confidential information. In addition, properly designed and monitored audit trails can enhance user accountability by detecting and recording unauthorized access to confidential information. CPRI has produced position papers on user authentication and access to patient data and provided substantive guidelines on security policies, security education programs, job descriptions for information security managers, model confidentiality policies, and security functionality requirements for CPR systems (CPRI, 1995a,b, 1996b,d). CPRI and the American Health Information Management Association have been instrumental in developing model policies and legislation regarding confidentiality and privacy. Public Law 104-191 establishes legal sanctions for wrongful disclosure of individually identifiable health information. It also calls on the secretary of Health and Human Services to provide detailed recommendations on privacy of health data and procedures and rules for authorized disclosure of such information. The recently revitalized National Committee on Vital and Health Statistics (NCVHS) advises the secretary on this and other standards related to health information. Federal legislation is necessary to overcome many of the inadequacies and inconsistencies between the state regulations and laws that are described in this report.

Whereas stringent security measures should be applied to protect the confidentiality of patient information, it is also in the patient's best interest for the CPR to be accessible for appropriate, legitimate uses by authorized users. The measures used to protect the confidentiality of patient data must not be so onerous that clinicians taking care of a patient do not have ready access to the patient's health data. This balance must be carefully crafted in the enabling legislation and policy standards, and enforceable through system security functions. In addition to clinicians, researchers, quality assessment professionals, and health care managers need access to aggregate data to continuously improve health and the delivery of health care. Most of the time, these secondary uses of data can be satisfied without access to individually identifiable information.

Costs and Benefits

Certainly, the cost of developing a CPR system remains a significant barrier, but this barrier has been offset at least in part by three trends. First, as CPR-related technologies continue to advance, greater performance can be obtained for equivalent costs. Second, as integrated delivery systems become more prevalent, the demand for CPR and related information systems will increase, thus reducing the risk to developers. Third, some federal funds have been made available (e.g., through NLM and AHCPR) to address specific development challenges associated with CPRs. The stability and level of federal funding in the future, however, are uncertain.

Much of the enthusiasm for the CPR is based on the belief that a CPR system will reduce the cost and improve the quality of care through the existence of better-informed health care providers and patients, the elimination of duplicate testing, and better coordination of treatment by more than one health care provider. Since the first edition, additional data have been published on the positive impact of CPR systems on the cost and quality of health care. As existing clinical systems continued to accumulate data, new studies have demonstrated improvements in the quality of care or reductions in the cost of care (Classen et al., 1991, 1992; Evans et al., 1992; Schoenbaum and Barnett, 1992; Tierney et al., 1993; Grandia et al., 1995). However, most of the carefully done empirical studies presented in the literature have examined the benefits of systems that are not commercially available. Like other enabling technologies (e.g., electronic mail, cellular telephones, computers), it may be difficult to identify and reliably quantify the direct and indirect benefits attributable to the CPR system. It is hard to quantify what is better, when so much may not even have been possible without the enabling technology.

Although discrete benefits of CPR system features have been quantified in selected environments, the comprehensive capital and operating costs have not been fully articulated. It is known, however, that the costs are substantial. One estimate for a capital budget (including capitalized labor costs) for an integrated health care information system with $1 billion to $2 billion in revenue is $75 million to $275 million (Council on Competitiveness, 1996). At a time when health care organizations need to reduce their costs, allocating capital to information systems is still a challenge. Although it is tempting to propose that large empirical studies be conducted to produce definitive cost-benefit data, it may be unrealistic to expect that such studies can be undertaken, or that they could truly represent the diverse health systems in the United States.

Many health care organizations are aware of the benefits of CPR systems, but have questions on how to implement and use this new technology. Recognizing that experience with these systems is not widespread, CPRI developed a program to help disseminate the knowledge of those who have previous experience with CPR systems and to provide a tool to help organizations undertake new projects and initiatives. Modeled after the Malcolm Baldrige Quality Award Program, CPRI developed a program to promote quality in CPR system projects. The program is named after Nicholas E. Davies, a member of the IOM Patient Record committee who was tragically killed in an airplane crash just as the committee was concluding its work. The Nicholas E. Davies Annual CPR Recognition Symposia provide recognition for organizations demonstrating exemplary measurable impact of CPR systems on health care at their organizations (CPRI, 1995c, 1996c, 1997).

The objectives of the Davies CPR Systems Recognition Program are to: (a) promote the vision of CPR systems through concrete examples, (b) provide visibility and recognition for excellence in CPR system implementation and demonstrated results, (c) provide a forum for discussing critical success factors and lessons learned, and (d) provide criteria for evaluating CPR system projects (CPRI, 1996a). A comprehensive set of evaluation criteria was developed in an iterative fashion by CPRI and external experts. Emphasizing the fact that successful CPR system projects require a comprehensive, multidisciplinary team approach led by senior management, the evaluation categories are divided into four categories: (1) management, (2) system functionality, (3) technology, and (4) impact on quality, costs, and access. These categories reflect the notion that a CPR system implementation project is more than a selection or development of an information system product, it is the conceptualization of a new recordkeeping system that efficiently and effectively supports the delivery of health care and health promotion by the health care team. Existing organizational structures, departmental cultures, and an inward focus may have to be transformed to efficiently deliver high-quality care and effectively compete for managed care contracts. The CPR system is an essential tool to accomplish these broader goals.

Leadership

Due to the barriers described above, leadership of and commitment to CPR system projects must come from the top of an organization. The organization's

Board of Directors must fund and support the implementation and use of CPR systems as a business imperative. Often, chief executive officers must act on personal conviction, existing evidence of benefits, and the desire to capitalize on a strategic differentiator—the value of data. In the new managed care market, a CPR system is not only an essential tool for health professionals, it is a business imperative. Time will tell whether investing in clinical systems provides a strategic advantage or is a minimum requirement to "stay in the game." Neither outcome favors continuing the status quo. It takes a combination of leadership conviction, organizational fiscal strength, and medical informatics and systems expertise to implement CPR systems effectively. Where such leadership exists, CPR systems are more likely to be acquired and successfully implemented.

CONCLUSION

A careful reading of *The Computer-Based Patient Record* by all stakeholders in health care is still fruitful. We believe that the original vision described by the IOM Committee on Improving the Patient Record was correct and remains timely and essential to the success of the new health care delivery system. Widespread use of CPRs would serve both private- and public-sector objectives to transform health care delivery in the United States. Equally important, early evidence indicates that the introduction and use of robust CPRs will enhance the health of citizens and reduce the costs of care, and in so doing, the use of CPRs will strengthen the nation's productivity.

Technological advances aside, progress toward CPRs as envisioned in this report has been slower than anticipated. The IOM committee expressed its strong belief that the early phase of CPRI's activities should be federally initiated and funded. A major coordinated national effort with federal funding and strong advisory support from the private sector is needed to accelerate the pace of change in the United States. Health care is a public good and many of the barriers to widespread implementation of CPR systems require national mandates, policy changes, or, in some cases, new legislation. Leadership in government and the private sector must be galvanized to make sweeping changes where possible (e.g., a national UHI, confidentiality legislation) and to instigate, motivate, and provide incentives to accelerate development of solutions to other impediments (e.g., terminology standards).

Data are the currency of quality management and the endowment for continuous quality improvement of patient care. Only by capturing primary clinical data from health care providers in a way that they can be applied to health care decisions for individuals and to policy decisions for populations can the United States achieve its goal of providing high-quality, affordable health care for all. A computer-based patient record is essential to accomplishing that goal.

ACKNOWLEDGMENTS

We are deeply indebted to Octo Barnett who refocused our attention on the important points we were trying to communicate. The message is far stronger because of his constructive comments. We thank Don Detmer and Elaine Steen for their gracious invitation to contribute to this second edition.

REFERENCES

Accredited Standards Committee X12N. Series of EDI standards available from Data Interchange Standards Association, Inc., 1800 Diagonal Road, Suite 200, Alexandria, VA 22314-2852.

ACR/NEMA Standards Publication. Digital Imaging and Communications in Medicine (DICOM). PS 3.1-3.13. National Electrical Manufactuers Assocation, 2102 L Street N.W., Washington, D.C. 1992-1995.

AMIA (American Medical Informatics Association) Board of Directors. 1994. Standards for Medical Identifiers, Codes, and Messages Needed to Create an Efficient Computer-Stored Medical Record. *Journal of the American Medical Informatics Association* 1:1-7.

ASTM Committee E-31 on Healthcare Informatics. Group of standards available from ASTM, 100 Barr Harbor Drive, West Conshohocken, PA 19428-2959.

Barnett, G. O. 1984. The application of computer-based medical-record systems in ambulatory practice. *New England Journal of Medicine* 310:1643-1650.

Barnett, G. O., J. J. Cimino, J. A. Hupp, and E. P. Hoffer. 1987. DXplain: An evolving diagnostic decision-support system. *Journal of the American Medical Association* 258:67-74.

Barrows, Jr., R. C., and P. D. Clayton. 1996. Privacy, confidentiality, and electronic medical records. *Journal of the American Medical Informatics Association* 3:139-148.

Berner, E. S., J. R. Jackson, and J. Algina. 1996. Relationships among performance scores of four diagnostic decision support systems. *Journal of the American Medical Informatics Association* 3:208-215.

Chute, C. G., S. P. Cohen, K. E. Campbell, D. E. Oliver, and J. R. Campbell. 1996. The content coverage of clinical classifications. *Journal of the American Medical Informatics Association* 3:224-231.

Cimino, J. J., S. A. Socratous, and P. D. Clayton. 1995. Internet as clinical information system: Application development using the World Wide Web. *Journal of the American Medical Association* 2:273-284.

Classen, D. C., R. S. Evans, S. L. Pestotnik, S. D. Horn, R. L. Menlove, and J. P. Burke. 1992. The timing of prophylactic administration of antibiotics and the risk of surgical-wound infection. *New England Journal of Medicine* 326:281-286.

Classen, D. C., S. L. Pestotnik, R. S. Evans, and J. P. Burke. 1991. Computerized surveillance of adverse drug events in hospital patients [published erratum appears in *Journal of the American Medical Association* 267(14):1922, 1992] [see comments]. *Journal of the American Medical Association* 266:2847-2851.

Council on Competitiveness. 1996. *Highway to Health: Transforming U.S. Health Care in the Information Age.* Washington, D.C.: Council on Competitiveness.

Covell, D. G., G. C. Uman, and P. R. Manning. 1985. Information needs in office practice: Are they being met? *Annals of Internal Medicine* 103:596-599.

CPRI (Computer-based Patient Record Institute). 1995a. *Guidelines for Establishing Information Security Policies at Organizations Using Computer-Based Patient Record Systems.* Schaumburg, Ill.: CPRI.

CPRI. 1995b. *Guidelines for Information Security Education Programs at Organizations Using Computer-Based Patient Record Systems.* Schaumburg, Ill.: CPRI.

CPRI. 1995c. *Proceedings of the First Annual Nicholas E. Davies CPR Recognition Symposium.* Ed. E. B. Steen. Schaumburg, Ill.: CPRI.

CPRI. 1996a. CPR Systems Evaluation Work Group: CPR Project Evaluation Criteria (version 2.1). The Nicholas E. Davies Recognition Program. Schaumburg, Ill.: CPRI.

CPRI. 1996b. *Guidelines for Managing Information Security Programs at Organizations Using Computer-Based Patient Record Systems.* Schaumburg, Ill.: CPRI.

CPRI. 1996c. *Proceedings of the Second Annual Nicholas E. Davies CPR Recognition Symposium.* Ed. E. B. Steen. Schaumburg, Ill.: CPRI.

CPRI. 1996d. *Sample Confidentiality Statements and Agreements for Organizations.* Schaumburg, Ill.: CPRI.

CPRI. 1997. *Proceedings of the Third Annual Nicholas E. Davies CPR Recognition Symposium.* Ed. J. J. Teich. Schaumburg, Ill.: CPRI.

Detmer, D. E., and E. B. Steen. 1996. Shoring up protection of personal health data. *Issues in Science and Technology* 12:73-78.

Evans, R. S., J. P. Burke, D. C. Classen, R. M. Gardner, R. L. Menlove, K. M. Goodrich, L. E. Stevens, and S. L. Pestotnik. 1992. Computerized identification of patients at high risk for hospital-acquired infections. *American Journal of Infectious Control* 20:4-10.

Feldman, M. J., and G. O. Barnett. 1991. An approach to evaluating the accuracy of DXplain. *Computational Methods and Programs in Biomedicine* 35:261-266.

Grandia, L. D., T. A. Pryor, D. F. Willson, R. M. Gardner, P. J. Haug, S. M. Huff, B. R. Farr, and S. H. Lam. 1995. Building a computer-based patient record in an evolving integrated health system. Pp. 5-33 in *Proceedings of the First Annual Nicholas E. Davies CPR Recognition Symposium,* ed. E. B. Steen. Schaumburg, Ill.: CPRI.

Hammond, W. E. 1984. The Status of Healthcare Standards in the United States. Pp. 87-92 in *Information Systems with Fading Boundaries,* ed. W. E. Hammond, A. R. Bakker, and M. J. Ball. New York: Elsevier Science.

Health Level Seven (HL-7), Version 2.2. 1994. Health Level Seven, 3300 Washtenaw Ave., Suite 227, Ann Arbor, MI 48104-4250. 1994.

Hoechst Marion Roussel, Inc. 1995. HMO-PPO Digest.

Hripcsak, G., P. D. Clayton, T. A. Pryor, P. Haug, O. B. Wigertz, and J. Van der Lei. 1990. The Arden syntax for medical logic modules. Pp. 200-204 in *Proceedings of the Fourteenth Symposium on Computer Applications in Medical Care.* Washington, D.C.: IEEE Computer Society Press.

Humphreys, B. L., W. T. Hole, A. T. McCray, and J. M. Fitzmaurice. 1996. Planned NLM/AHCPR large-scale vocabulary test: Using UMLS technology to determine the extent to which controlled vocabularies cover terminology needed for health care and public health. *Journal of the American Medical Informatics Association* 3:281-287.

IEEE (Institute of Electrical and Electronics Engineers). 1995. Standards available from IEEE Standards Department, 445 Hoes Lane, PO Box 1331, Piscataway, NJ 08855-1331.

IOM (Institute of Medicine). 1993. *Assessing Health Care Reform.* Washington, D.C.: National Academy Press.

Johnson, M. E., K. B. Langton, R. B. Haynes, and A. Mathieu. 1994. Effects of computer-based clinical decision support systems on clinician performance and patient outcome: A critical appraisal. *Annals of Internal Medicine* 120:135-142.

Lindberg, D. A. B. 1995. The High-Performance Computing and Communications Program, the national information infrastructure, and health care. *Journal of the American Medical Informatics Association* 2:156-159.

McDonald, C. J. 1976. Protocol-based computer reminders, the quality of care, and the non-perfectibility of man. *New England Journal of Medicine* 295:1351-1355.

McDonald, C. J., S. L. Hui, D. M. Smith, et al. 1984. Reminders to physicians from an introspective computer medical record: A two-year randomized trial. *Annals of Internal Medicine* 100:130-138.

Miller, R., F. E. Masarie, and J. D. Myers. 1986. Quick medical reference (QMR) for diagnostic assistance. *MD Computing* 3:34-48.

NCPDP (National Council for Prescription Drug Programs). 1992. Standards available from NCPDP, 4201 North 24th St, Suite 365, Phoenix, AZ 85016.

NRC (National Research Council). 1996. *The Unpredictable Uncertainty: Information Infrastructure Through 2000.* Washington, D.C.: National Academy Press.

National Committee for Quality Assurance. 1997. *A Road Map for Information Systems: Evolving Systems to Support Performance Measurement.* National Committee for Quality Assurance.

Schoenbaum, S. C., and G. O. Barnett. 1992. Automated ambulatory medical records systems: An orphan technology. *International Journal of Technical Assessment in Health Care* 8:598-609.

Shortliffe, E. H., H. L. Bleich, C. G. Caine, D. R. Masys, and D. W. Simborg. 1996. The federal role in the health information infrastructure: A debate of the pros and cons of government intervention. *Journal of the American Medical Informatics Association* 3:249-257.

Sittig, D. F., and W. W. Stead. 1994. Computer-based physician order entry: The state of the art. *Journal of the American Medical Informatics Association* 1:108-123.

Sullivan, F., and E. Mitchell. 1995. Has general practitioner computing made a difference to patient care? A systematic review of published reports. *British Medical Journal* 311:848-852.

Tang, P. C., and V. L. Patel. 1994. Major issues in user interface design for health professional workstations: Summary and recommendations. *International Journal of Biomedical Computing* 34:139-148.

Tang, P. C., D. Fafchamps, and E. H. Shortliffe. 1994. Traditional medical records as a source of clinical data in the outpatient setting. Pp. 575-579 in *Proceedings of the Eighteenth Symposium on Computer Applications in Medical Care,* ed. J. G. Ozbolt. Washington, D.C.

Tang, P. C., M. A. Jaworski, C. A. Fellencer, N. Kreider, M. P. LaRosa, and W. C. Marquardt. 1996. Clinician information activities in diverse ambulatory care practices. Pp. 12-16 in *Proceedings of the 1996 AMIA Annual Fall Symposium,* ed. J. J. Cimino. Washington, D.C.: American Medical Informatics Association.

Tierney, W. M., C. J. McDonald, D. K. Martin, and M. P. Rogers. 1987. Computerized display of past test results. Effect on outpatient testing. *Annals of Internal Medicine* 107:569-574.

Tierney, W. M., M. E. Miller, and C. J. McDonald. 1990. The effect on test ordering of informing physicians of the charges for outpatient diagnostic tests [see comments]. *New England Journal of Medicine* 322:1499-1504.

Tierney, W. M., M. E. Miller, J. M. Overhage, and C. J. McDonald. 1993. Physician inpatient order writing on microcomputer workstations: Effects on resource utilization. *Journal of the American Medical Association* 269:379-383.

Tierney, W. M., J. M. Overhage, B. Y. Takesue, L. E. Harris, M. D. Murray, D. L. Vargo, and C. J. McDonald. 1995. Computerizing guidelines to improve care and patient outcomes: The example of heart failure. *Journal of the American Medical Informatics Association* 2:316-322.

Commentary

A Progress Report on Computer-Based Patient Records in Europe

Jan H. van Bemmel, Astrid M. van Ginneken, and Johan van der Lei

After more than two decades of pioneering efforts, in both the United States and Europe, a new era in the use of computer-stored patient data has clearly begun. The proliferation of inexpensive personal computers and workstations, the development of more user-friendly interfaces, the standardization of network technology, the original release of this report 6 years ago, and the stimulation of health care telematics (i.e., network communications) in Europe have contributed significantly to this growing interest. Equally important, developers of systems have acquired much experience since they first attempted to develop electronic patient records, and their subsequent attempts have become more successful and gained momentum.

In this commentary we discuss some recent developments in computer-based patient records (CPRs) in Europe and review some CPR developments in Europe that fall within the Framework Programs on Research and Development of the European Union. Specifically, we review European developments in CPRs for primary care, clinical care (i.e., hospital care), and shared care. We also address the use of CPR data beyond patient care and two barriers to CPR development: protection of patient confidentiality and standards development for data.

THE CURRENT STATE OF CPRs IN EUROPE

Computer-based information systems are now abundant in a large percentage of European hospitals as well as in primary care settings. Systems support general tasks such as patient administration, scheduling, and billing, as well as specific tasks such as in the clinical laboratory, radiology, or the catheterization laboratory. Hospital information systems are primarily administration oriented

and seldom contain patient record data other than, for example, laboratory results, drug prescriptions, or diagnostic codes. Some systems store patient data,
but none of them fully replaces the paper-based patient record. Many existing
systems are not connected or are only loosely interconnected in networks. CPRs
are being developed as part of a hospitalwide network (Degoulet et al., 1991; Van
Mulligen et al., 1994; Scherrer et al., 1995) or as stand-alone or interconnected
applications, such as in primary care (Westerhof et al., 1987; Branger et al., 1992;
van der Lei et al., 1993). Increasingly, systems are being interconnected by electronic data interchange.

The field of hospital information systems in Europe consists, on the one hand,
of mainly homemade systems (e.g., Bakker, 1984; Scherrer et al., 1995) sometimes supporting a group of hospitals and, on the other, of systems offered
by industry, mainly of U.S. origin. A wide variety of information systems are
operational on different platforms. Information systems in Europe reflect the differences in health care organizations which arise from the different historical
developments, legislation, education, and languages among European countries.
Therefore, systems developed in one European country are rarely installed in
another country. This is also why the European hospital information system industry, with few exceptions, is virtually absent from the global market.

The differences in health care structures of different European countries
might pose less of a problem for patient-centered approaches, such as CPRs. In
all countries, patient care itself is quite similar. Europe has succeeded early at its
attempts at CPR development and has since made considerable progress in the
use of CPRs, especially in the primary care setting (van der Lei et al., 1991a;
Millman et al., 1995). On the basis of these successes, several collaborative
projects were started in health care; these were financially subsidized in part by
the European Union (EU, 1994). Three developments related to CPRs in Europe
deserve attention: the use of CPRs in the primary care setting, in hospitals, and
for shared care (i.e., collaboration between care providers). In addition, in the
area of standardization in health care, the European Union plays a pivotal role on
a global scale as well (De Moor, 1993).

Network technology and communication (in Euope the latter is called
telematics) are now prominent developments in information technology and have
a large impact on health care (Branger et al., 1992; EU, 1994). By using standard
communication networks and standard software (De Moor, 1993), data interchange between the four levels of health care delivery (i.e., the region, the institution, the clinical department or outpatient clinic, and the individual physician,
nurse, or patient) is more efficient. A fully operational exchange of patient data
between systems, with proper authorization, is one of the present challenges in
Euopean health care.

The data in CPRs are not begging to be used for electronic data exchange,
resarch, and shared care. The use of CPRs for purposes other than direct patient
care has been associated with several problems (van der Lei et al., 1991a; Vlug

and van der Lei, 1995). These limitations are, for instance, the lack of a common terminology for patient data collection, or the use of different modes for the CPR systems. As the knowledge gained from experience accumulates, CPR developers learn important lessons, particularly the need to develop structured patient records based on a clear conceptual model. If CPR systems are not based on a conceptual model, and if the data in CPRs are not well structured, it will not be possible to use CPR data for different goals, nor will it be possible for such data to be exchanged between health care providers to support shared care. Therefore, if CPR systems are to be used for these other goals, care providers should realize that it is not sufficient that the systems merely support their own practice or clinic, but they should take care that patient data can be exchanged over the entire health care domain and be used, for instance, to support clinical research, decision-making, the assessment of the quality of care, or management and planning.

A variety of CPR applications and projects have been completed or are ongoing including those supported through Framework Programs on Research and Development of the European Union. They concern computer-based records for primary care, in hospitals, and for shared care, as well as the use of data in CPRs for research, assessment of the quality of care, and decision support. Other projects focus on what the Institute of Medicine (IOM) Committee on Improving the Patient Record classified as barriers to CPR development: privacy and confidentiality and standardization of terminologies and data-exchange formats.

Several developments related to CPRs in Europe are discussed below, including the status of CPRs in the primary care settings, in hospitals, and in shared care (i.e., collaboration between care providers). The final sections consider more specific uses of CPR data and remaining barriers to wider use of the computer-based patient record.

CPR SYSTEMS IN PRIMARY CARE

In some European countries, especially The Netherlands (van der Lei et al., 1993) and the United Kingdom (Millman et al., 1995), there has been a rapid increase in the use of information systems by general practitioners (GPs) in primary care (Figure 1). CPRs are incorporated into these information systems and are quickly replacing existing paper-based records. The use of CPRs by GPs in particular is rapidly increasing. At the beginning of 1996 it was estimated that more than 90 percent of all GPs in The Netherlands and the United Kingdom used information systems in their practices. About 50 percent of Dutch GPs had implemented a CPR system for the support of patient care and about 25 percent of GPs had a paperless office.

Similar figures apply to the United Kingdom (Millman et al., 1995). This is directly related to the fact that in both the United Kingdom and The Netherlands, GPs are the "gatekeepers" in health care. Most GPs run a practice by themselves or with a small number of colleagues. In contrast, specialists work in large insti-

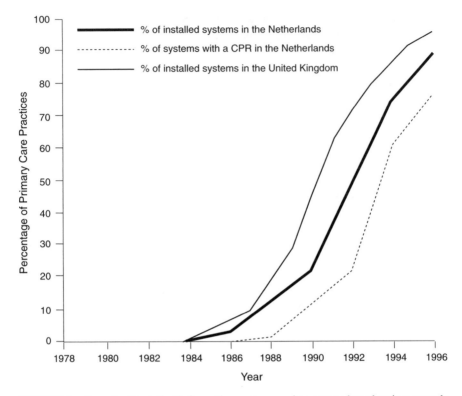

FIGURE 1 Growth of installed information systems and computer-based patient records in primary care in The Netherlands (100% represents 6,500 general practitioners [GPs]) and England and Wales (where 100% represents 9,000 GPs) as a function of time. The values for 1996 are extrapolations. Not indicated is the growing number of primary care systems that are electronically connected to other health care systems (see also the text and Figure 3).

tutions in more complex settings, involving many more departments and personnel. Furthermore, GPs keep less extensive records so that data entry is less time-consuming and less detailed.

The actual situation in The Netherlands offers a good example of both the success and the potential use of CPRs (van der Lei et al., 1993). This can be attributed to four factors: (1) the role of GPs, (2) physician training, (3) the structure of health care, and (4) population-based care.

Role of GPs

From the outset, professional organizations of GPs have played an active role in setting guidelines for information systems in general practice and in assessing the systems available in the market. This active role was started in the early 1980s, when they identified the basic needs of GPs for using systems in their practices and set the first broad guidelines for systems tailored specifically for primary care. Furthermore, these organizations announced to industry that they would recommend to their members that they use only those systems that would meet their requirements. In this way, a de facto standard was established. Since then, systems requirements are refined and extended every 2 to 3 years, and vendors must submit their systems for reevaluation by professional organizations. This iterative way of refining guidelines and assessing systems gives potential buyers of systems a basis on which to judge the available information systems. It also gives vendors clear-cut standards for their products. During the last 15 years, the definition of standards started with requirements for patient administration and evolved into standards for diagnostic coding (in all systems the International Classification for Primary Care has been implemented [Lamberts and Wood, 1987]), drug prescriptions (all systems use the same national thesaurus for drugs), and the type of data to be contained in a basic CPR and requirements for electronically interchanging patient data between different systems in the primary care setting, that is, from one GP's system to that of another.

Training

The success of information systems is largely determined by physicians' expectations. Education at medical faculties of universities prepares physicians in the use of computer-based information systems and patient records. Early on, students get acquainted with how to use computers for the documentation of patient data in CPRs. Professional organizations have also ensured that postgraduate training of GPs conveys a realistic set of expectations. These expectations must be realistic, because if they are too high they lead to disillusionment, and if they are too low they may impede the introduction of systems. The training emphasizes that the proper use of systems and CPRs reduces administrative workload, increases the accuracy of billing (no accountable patient data are lost), and enables the production of referral letters, the use of electronic data interchange, and the tracking of certain categories of patients.

Potential users should realize that, certainly at the beginning, investments must be made. The investments must be expressed not only in financial terms but also in time and personal efforts. For instance, for a typical practice of about 2,300 patients, it takes about 2 years for all patient data to be entered into the system's CPR. This data transcription from paper to computer is most often done at the time that patients come for a consultation, since the majority of patients pay a visit to their GP once every 2 years. A GP who is just starting to use a CPR system needs an extra 2 to 3 minutes during the consultation. The GP's assistant enters data related to all administrative operations, such as patient admission and patient scheduling, but the GP enters the patient care-related data into the CPR.

Structure of Health Care

The factors described above are related to the role and training of GPs in using CPRs and may be useful for other countries. A third factor, however, is strongly related to the structure of health care in The Netherlands, which in many ways is comparable to that in the United Kingdom and Scandinavian countries. Patients in The Netherlands and the United Kingdom have a single GP who coordinates their health care, acting as a gatekeeper to other specialists; the latter report back to the GP. Several projects are now under way to use electronic data interchange for this GP-specialist communication (see the section on "CPR Systems for Shared Care," page 32). Thus, in principle, the GP coordinates the health care-related data for a single patient over the patient's lifetime and is requested by other specialists to share that information. The GP's role as coordinator eases the introduction of CPR systems because the demands of care are easier to meet when the data are available in electronic form. This factor may be increasingly relevant in the United States as managed care and capitated reimbursement continue to penetrate the health care delivery market.

Population-Based Care

A fourth reason for the success of the acceptance of CPRs in the primary care setting is the fact that Dutch general practice is population-based care, in contrast to institution- or physician-based care. The Dutch primary care system can be characterized as providing services that are responsive to the needs both of the individual patients and the population at large. Such a population-based orientation creates demands that are easier to satisfy when CPRs are introduced. For instance, CPRs with properly coded data greatly facilitate the creation of a gender-age register to report on statistics in primary care or active case finding (e.g., for periodic cervical smears or cardiovascular risk assessments). The availability of CPRs facilitates studies on the use and effects of drugs in the population and postmarketing drug surveillance (see the section on "Use of CPR Data," page 34).

CPR SYSTEMS IN HOSPITALS

Electronic information technology has been introduced in all hospitals in Europe. This is no longer restricted to special areas of care, such as radiology or the laboratory. In principle, the available technology allows central and monolithic hospital information systems to be transformed into hospitalwide networks with "intelligent" workstations or personal computers throughout the hospital, from the consultation room to close to the bedside. This transformation is just beginning, however. At present, graphical workstations and network technology are the latest developments in the computer industry. Client-server protocols ease the integration of systems and distribution of processing tasks (Degoulet et al., 1991; Van Mulligen et al., 1994; Nowlan et al., 1994). In principle, workstations offer an environment in which, from the user's perspective, all applications running either locally or through a network act as a single integrated system. Several institutions are developing health care workstations that enable the integration of patient data scattered throughout different systems (Degoulet et al., 1991; Van Mulligen et al., 1994; van Bemmel et al., 1996a). In principle, such systems offer to the clinician on one computer screen patient data, images, and biological signals, regardless of the computer on which they are stored or the system on which they are processed.

Yet, although the technical issues involved in the integration of various systems were slowly being solved, the absence of a conceptual model for a CPR was increasingly becoming a stumbling block, particularly as the amount of available data increased. Thus emerged a trend in which a technical infrastructure (the platform for the CPR) takes care of the communication with the numerous systems available in the hospital, including legacy systems, such as a laboratory system, a picture archiving and communication system (PACS), or an electrocardiogram (ECG) interpretation system. CPRs are developed at the core of this integration platform. This distinction is not trivial. When developing the platforms, questions such as how an existing legacy system should be embedded are addressed on a technical level. On the level of CPR development, questions relate, for example, to how the data will be presented to the user in a consistent manner or what additional data the physician must record are addressed.

Platforms for CPRs

Both the Helios (Degoulet at al., 1991) and the Hermes (Van Mulligen et al., 1994) integrated clinical workstations offer an environment for systems integration. Communication between applications is automatically performed by the workstation and follows ISO[1] standards (ISO, 1987). Instead of having one large central database of patient data, all existing databases and applications are left unchanged and patient data are combined by the workstation on demand. This has two advantages over one large integrated database. First, data can remain distributed and stored at places that are most convenient (i.e., close to where the data are collected and used). Second, commercially available applications can be used for data processing without modifying them.

The Hermes workstation was initially developed to support clinical data analysis, but its architecture has also been extended to support patient care. It is

---

[1]ISO: International Standards Organization.

integrated with the generic CPR system ORCA[2] (van Ginneken, 1996). Hermes is also able to integrate with legacy systems by encapsulation.

The Helios workstation, similar to Hermes in many respects, also integrates alphanumeric data (text), images, and biological signals. The Helios platform is being used as one of the building blocks of a new generation of hospital information systems. The Hermes approach, originally developed on a Unix platform, has now migrated to a Windows NT/95 environment, forming the basis for the European project I4C (van Bemmel et al., 1996), as explained below.

Integrated CPRs

As an example of the introduction of a CPR in a clinical department, we briefly describe the European project I4C (Integration and Communication for the Continuity of Cardiac Care). Although I4C is intended to support cardiology, it uses a generic CPR, ORCA, which is also applicable to other departments. In this way, the CPR used in the I4C project can be used by many other clinical departments (van Ginneken et al., 1995; van Ginnekin and Stam, 1995), because it contains a variety of patient data: patient history, physical examination findings, laboratory test results, images, biological signals, and so forth. Real-time data, such as from the catheterization laboratory, are also intended to be incorporated into the CPR. Data are meant to be used by more than one physician (e.g., the cardiologist often must coordinate his or her treatment with that of other specialists in the hospital or with GPs in primary care).

Figure 2 presents the CPR structure that forms the basis for the I4C project, together with its branches to other systems in the hospital or elsewhere. Patient record data, as well as images such as echocardiograms and coronary angiograms, or signals such as ECGs or blood pressure curves are collected, stored, and presented by using the workstation.

The I4C project in principle is intended to support cardiac care, from prevention and treatment to follow-up and rehabilitation. This is accomplished by: (a) consistently recording patient data in the CPR; (b) accessing diagnostic and therapeutic information; (c) accessing patient data, images, and biological signals wherever they are stored and irrespective of where the inquiry originates; and (d) collecting well-defined reference sets of patient data.

---

[2]ORCA (Open Record for patient CAre) is a generic CPR system in which the knowledge model consists of a predefined vocabulary and knowledge about how the terms of that vocabulary may be combined into meaningful expressions (van Ginneken, 1996). ORCA is used in the framework of different (European) projects (van Bemmel et al., 1996). ORCA contains a powerful model for structuring a CPR and a knowledge model for capturing patient data. Moreover, because it is generic, ORCA can be used for different areas of health care and is user-adaptable. The relationships between the terms in the knowledge model are semantically defined (van Ginneken et al., 1993, Moorman et al., 1994), for instance, in an acyclic directed graph.

Data are to be used not only for patient care, research, and education but also for the assessment of the quality of care and for management and planning. The fourth issue is similar to the data collection that resulted from the European CSE[3] project that preceded I4C (Willems et al., 1991). The project is carried out by centers in The Netherlands—which provides coordination—the United Kingdom, France, Germany, Italy, and Greece.

CPR Data Entry

For a CPR to have benefits, the data in that record need to be structured and coded, at least to a certain degree. Obtaining structured and coded data, however, has proved to be a significant hurdle. Physicians are accustomed to paper records. How physicians use these records has been the subject of several European projects (e.g., Nygren and Henriksson, 1992). From such investigations it became apparent that physicians are far more likely to use computers to consult the data in present patient records than to enter patient data. This is not surprising: Data entry requires more effort from the physician than browsing through the record. Some researchers have argued that direct input by physicians will have to wait for radical improvements of the human-machine interface, such as speech input. Experience in a number of countries where GPs are particularly using CPRs (e.g., The Netherlands, the United Kingdom, and Sweden) has shown, however, that physicians will accept the limitations of the current human-machine interaction.

Views of CPR data for patient care, decision support, scientific data analysis, or assessment of quality of care require patient data to be highly structured and unambiguous. It is difficult to fulfill these requirements with narrative (textual) data (e.g., Moorman et al., 1994). Ideally, therefore, patient data should be acquired directly from the physician in a structured format and, preferably, should also be entered by the physician. To accomplish this, different approaches to data entry have received attention: form-driven data entry, natural language processing, and structured data entry. The last two methods are also the focus of several research projects in Europe (Nowlan and Rector, 1991; Baud et al., 1992; Moorman et al., 1994).

Natural Language Processing

Natural language processing intends to automatically extract coded medical data from free text. European research in this area has mainly been done by Baud and colleagues in Geneva (1992). The basic advantage of natural language processing is that physicians do not have to alter the way in which they express their findings or document their decisions. Only when its application domain is strictly

---

[3]CSE: Common standards for quantitative electrocardiography.

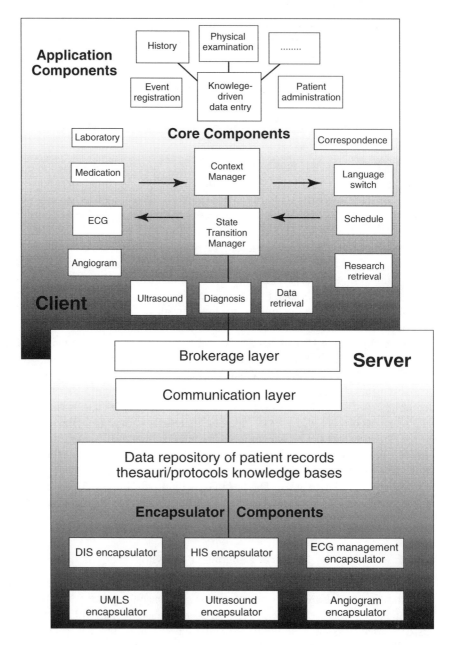

confined can natural language processing offer advantages. A fundamental disadvantage of natural language processing is that the data-capturing process itself cannot be influenced and improved. Data that the physician has not written or spoken remain unknown. Freedom of expression is inherent to free text (Moorman et al., 1994). Therefore, it is difficult to impose structure on data that are used as input for natural language processing.

Structured Data Entry

Another way of data entry is context sensitive and is adaptable to different clinical domains. It is called structured data entry and consists of forms whose content is knowledge driven. In a structured data entry-oriented European project, the forms are structured, but their contents can continuously be adapted to accommodate the user's requirements and personal preferences (Moorman et al., 1994). In addition to a knowledge model, it contains a predefined vocabulary and specifications on how the terms of the vocabulary may be combined into meaningful expressions. The knowledge base keeps track of the individual physician's definitions of expressions with a nontrivial meaning, such as "the heart is normal" or "gastroenteritis complaints." When such expressions are used for the first time, the system will prompt the physician-user for an explicit description. Upon later use of such expressions, the system will store its explicit substitute. In this way, efficiency and completeness can be reconciled.

Structured data entry is also an efficient tool for enhancing data completeness and testing for data reliability (Whiting-O'Keefe et al., 1985; Wyatt, 1994).

FIGURE 2 Example of the integration of a computer-based patient record (CPR) (ORCA; van Ginneken, 1996) in a clinical network of information systems being developed in the European project I4C (van Bemmel et al., 1996), in which centers from six countries collaborate. At the core of the CPR (called the client here) are three generic core components: the state transition manager, the context manager, and knowledge-driven data entry. The first two deal with all data acquisition, storage, and presentation and communication with the application components of the CPR system and the legacy systems elsewhere in the hospital. Communication is controlled by a brokerage layer and a communication layer, which are part of a group of servers. The broker follows protocols such as those agreed upon by the Common Object Request Broker Architecture (CORBA) Group (OMG, 1996); the communication layer provides data exchange via Electronic Data Interchange for Finance, Administration, Commerce, and Trade (EDIFACT) or HL-7. In the data repository, CPR data and knowledge bases are stored, together with coding systems and thesauruses for diagnoses and drugs. The six systems at the bottom are examples of "legacy systems" from which data (e.g., from a departmental or hospital information system), images (e.g., from an angiogram server), or biological signals (e.g., from an ECG management system) are to be transported to the CPR for presentation or processing. Integration with the legacy systems is provided by encapsulation (Van Mulligen et al., 1994).

Graphics and voice input may also serve to enhance the capabilities of structured data entry.

CPR SYSTEMS FOR SHARED CARE

An environment in which patient record data can be electronically interchanged regionally (Figure 3) is a necessary condition for a shared care environment (Branger et al., 1992, 1994; Branger and Duisterhout, 1995). Local and regional networks are increasingly used for the exchange of patient data between health care institutions. They are also used for communication with, for example, health insurance bodies, governmental organizations, libraries, and research institutions. Orders and payments are exchanged by electronic data interchange, databases are consulted remotely, and laboratory data or referral letters are mailed electronically. Communication between specialists and GPs is also increasingly taking place via telecommunication. In some instances specialists and general practitioners communicate directly with a patient in the patient's home, for example, patients with pacemakers, undergoing hemodialysis, or receiving palliative care. For some purposes, remote medical consultation (telemedicine) is also envisaged. Several regional shared-care networks are under development in Europe within the Framework Programs for Research and Development in health care telematics, as will be discussed below. Such regional networks are a logical extension of networks within hospitals.

With the existence of a computer-based shared care environment, new applications for patient-centered care have arisen, such as:

1. GPs are able to send a patient's data to the hospital to obtain results or diagnostic advice instead of referring the patient.

2. Patients' hospital stays are shorter and specialists may offer teleconsultation services.

3. Outpatient clinics increasingly function as diagnostic screening and ambulatory care centers. Patients are referred to these clinics only when specific diagnostic tests or interventions must be performed.

4. Patient admission and scheduling are greatly facilitated, resulting in better planning and decreased waiting times for examinations.

In the next two sections we provide two examples of European projects involving the use of CPR data for shared care. The first describes the project CoCo, concerning the coordination and continuity of health care (Bernstein and Jensen, 1994). The second describes a project that deals with the exchange of data in health care by smart cards, in this case, Diabcard (Schaefer and Sembritzki, 1996).

GP

Regional
Electronic
Data
Interchange

GP

Hospital

GP

Radiology   Pathology   Pharmacy   Laboratory

FIGURE 3   Regional electronic data-interchange network to support shared care. General practitioners (GPs) in primary care are interconnected with other health care providers, such as the clinical laboratory, pharmacies, pathology laboratories, radiology departments, and departments in the hospital. Usually, such an electronic data-interchange network makes use of public telephone lines or special lines (e.g., ISDN). In Europe, growing numbers of such networks are in development as part of European projects, such as the CoCo project (see text).

CoCo

The intention of the European project CoCo (Coordination and Continuity in Health Care) is to establish large-scale interconnected regional health care information networks, with the purpose of improving the coordination and continuity of health care (Bernstein and Jensen, 1994; van Bemmel et al., 1996). It uses available CPR-based systems and telecommunication infrastructures in the participating countries, European EDIFACT[4] standards, and electronic mail techniques. The project will not interfere with regional regulations and will not impose new rules on the users of the networks. A major effort is dedicated to ensuring that the project will be implemented in a coordinated and standard way. The practical guidelines and the experiences with the collaboration within CoCo should also be usable for other applications in Europe. CoCo has two goals:

1. Establishment of networks for the regional exchange of health care information. Each region will establish running networks that will allow for communication between all the major actors in health care: GPs, laboratories, radiology departments, hospitals, pharmacies, regional and national authorities, and social services and home care providers.

---

[4]EDIFACT: Electronic Data Interchange for Finance, Administration, Commerce, and Trade.

2. Establishment of links between the regions through CoCo Link. Coco Link ensures coordination between the regions to facilitate a common methodology, to start concerted developments, and to use standardized communication in all regions. For instance, it will provide guidelines, it is responsible for developing an electronic test bed that can be used to test EDIFACT solutions, and it will also establish networks between networks.

Many countries within the European Union, such as Denmark (coordination), The Netherlands, the United Kingdom, Ireland, Spain, and Greece, participate in CoCo. There is also an extension to Canada. A typical application within CoCo is shared care provided to patients with breast cancer. In this setting, GPs in primary care, internists, surgeons, and radiotherapists in secondary care collaborate with nurses in home care, covering the entire period from the first patient visit to the GP up to chemotherapy or surgery and, eventually, palliative care. All care providers have access to the same CPR; nurses in the home care setting use portable computers to exchange data with the system in the clinic.

Diabcard

In Germany, health insurance cards are regulated by law. During 1993 and 1994, more than 70 million smart cards (chip cards) were issued to German citizens, and about 165,000 read-write stations were installed in, for instance, practices, hospitals, and emergency rooms. The insurance cards are primarily used for administrative purposes, but debate is ongoing about the use of these smart cards as carriers of patient data. The German project Diabcard, which has also been extended to other European countries, uses smart cards for the storage and exchange of data for patients suffering from diabetes (Schaefer and Sembritzki, 1996). Other projects, such as for patients with cancer, are also being introduced in the German health care system. Standardization of the health care data on such cards is of utmost importance.

USE OF CPR DATA

Once patient data are available from CPRs in primary care centers and hospitals, the data can be harvested. We briefly discuss here a project dealing with critiquing a physician's care (van der Lei et al., 1991; van der Lei and Musen, 1991; van Bemmel, 1993). Another European project intends to integrate treatment protocols with CPR systems. It is oriented toward the support of clinical oncology. The third project deals with the assessment of care by using large collections of CPR data harvested from operational CPR systems in the primary care setting. This project is directed toward the postmarketing surveillance of drugs (Vlug and van der Lei, 1995).

Critiquing a Physician's Care

Automated review of CPRs is expected to limit errors in the delivery of care and to control costs. Two projects, carried out with GPs in The Netherlands, have investigated whether CPRs contain sufficient information to support direct care by assessing CPR data and generating critiques and decision support. In the first project (HyperCritic [van der Lei et al., 1991; van der Lei and Musen, 1991]), a system of critiquing the treatment of hypertension was developed. The second project (AsthmaCritic [Kuilboer and van der Lei, 1997]) covers the area of chronic obstructive respiratory diseases. Both systems rely on CPRs for patient data. HyperCritic was assessed in a research project, and we summarize here some of the main outcomes (van der Lei et al., 1991).

The critiquing systems generate comments in two stages. First, CPR data are automatically interpreted to review the actions of the GP at a given visit (e.g., starting a new drug, continuing treatment with a drug, or replacing one drug with another). Second, each action is assessed. The system searches the CPR for conditions that contraindicate that action (e.g., contraindications to specific drugs), determines whether the preparations required for the action have been performed, determines whether the GP has performed the routine monitoring required by the action, and searches for any undesirable condition that might have resulted from the action. Review of the CPR requires detailed knowledge of drugs, such as customary dosages, contraindications, side effects, interactions, workup requirements, and criteria for judging the efficacy of the treatment. Computer-based critiquing of patient care was compared with peer review-based critiquing in the area of mild hypertension. The comparisons revealed the following:

1. Automated assessment of CPR data by the computer-based critiquing system could compete successfully with peer review.

2. The system was not able to reproduce some comments of experts. This was the result of insufficient CPR data, the lack of sufficient medical consensus, or omissions in the knowledge base of the critiquing system.

On the basis of the outcomes of this and other studies reported in the literature, the following can be concluded:

1. Systems for the assessment of patient care should be able to acquire patient data automatically from the CPR.

2. Ideally, the care assessment system should be functionally integrated with the CPR system.

INTEGRATION OF PROTOCOLS WITH CPR SYSTEMS

In many patient care areas, protocols are used to increase both the efficiency and the quality of care. In principle, such protocols are not limited to certain hospitals, regions, or countries. This was the reason for starting a large European project on the use of protocols in health care (both in the clinic and in the primary care setting) called Prompt (Lagouarde et al., 1996; van Bemmel et al., 1996), which was based on the earlier European project Dilemma (Thomson, 1995). The project has been established by centers from the United Kingdom (which performs the coordination), France, and The Netherlands and intends to integrate these protocols with CPRs and to deliver and evaluate a set of tools for supporting the use of protocols. The initial focus of the project is oncology; this is now followed by a focus on the primary care and shared care settings.

The clinical objective is to install systems for supporting the treatment of cancer in specialty hospitals in the participating countries. Applications will be based on state-of-the-art therapeutic protocols. By the end of the project it is anticipated that the technology should be ready to be installed in centers in other countries as well. The following are other objectives of Prompt:

1. extensions to each hospital system, to support GPs, interconnected by regional networks for shared care;
2. initiation of comprehensive studies of the effects of the protocols on clinical outcomes; and
3. generic versions of the protocols for other clinical disciplines.

Review of CPR Databases

It is expected that CPRs will increasingly be used to improve the quality of care in practices, departments, and institutions as well as, for instance, to support postmarketing surveillance studies. Pressure from law enforcement bodies, third-party payers, peer-review organizations, hospitals, and physicians and patients themselves may lead to this use of automated review of CPRs. We briefly discuss a large ongoing project on the assessment of drug prescriptions in the population (Vlug and van der Lei, 1995; Visser et al., 1996). The project that is reported runs in The Netherlands, but similar projects have been started in other European countries (e.g., Germany and the United Kingdom).

Postmarketing surveillance examines the beneficial and adverse side effects of drugs on human health from the time that these drugs are marketed. Postmarketing surveillance consists of two stages: a hypothesis generation stage in which an effect or side effect is suspected and a hypothesis verification stage in which the hypothesis is tested. Hypothesis generation is typically based on the spontaneous reporting of potential side effects by physicians. Studies have indicated, however, that this spontaneous reporting leaves much to be desired. For instance, Classen and colleagues (1991) studied the prescription of drugs in cases in which the drug prescription was changed, increased, or stopped. It was shown that computerized monitoring of adverse drug events in hospitals by using computer-stored patient data offers many advantages over the voluntary reporting of such events.

An extensive project that analyzes prescriptions in primary care to support the postmarketing surveillance of drugs is under way in The Netherlands. To test a hypothesis, large populations need to be monitored. Reports of patient contacts with GPs are anonymously sent to a research database. The data in that database are subsequently used to conduct postmarketing surveillance studies (Vlug and van der Lei, 1995). The Dutch authorities responsible for drug safety are investigating the potential use of this type of database. Preliminary results indicate that the CPRs can be used as a way to track large numbers of patients and that use of CPRs will allow researchers to build longitudinal databases (Visser et al., 1996). At the end of 1996, about 250,000 patients were followed longitudinally; this number will increase to about 1.5 million in the next few years.

ADDRESSING BARRIERS

Privacy and Confidentiality

Now that CPR data are becoming available for the different goals mentioned in the introduction to this commentary, it is of great importance to protect these data, to guard the privacy of patients, and to protect the professional interests of health care providers (van Bemmel, 1992; Barber et al., 1996). Many parties (employers, insurance companies, etc.) are interested in permanent patient data,[5] and these data should be extremely well protected in CPR systems. In Europe there may be more sensitivity toward the improper use of patient data than elsewhere; this sensitivity could even impede the introduction of CPRs in some countries, and for some purposes could hamper the use of CPR data for goals other than patient care. In the different European countries, privacy laws control health care data, but privacy laws also exist in Europe as a whole. European law supersedes the laws of the individual countries. The right to privacy has been anchored in the *Treaty for the Protection of Human Rights and Fundamental Freedom*

---

[5]Medical data can be categorized into permanent data (e.g., one's genetic profile) and variable data (e.g., a blood pressure). The privacy aspect of permanent data is perhaps the most crucial. Generally, these two types of data are used in different ways: variable medical data (including alphanumeric data, biological signals, and pictures) are primarily used for the diagnosis and treatment of transient diseases, whereas permanent data are often strongly related to an individual's life and may possibly predict his or her future health. The latter category is also of interest for one's next of kin: parents, brothers, sisters, and children. Genetic data, for instance, do not change or age; they are valid for an entire lifetime.

(Treaty of Rome, 1954) and in European law (EU, 1995). Yet, it will be difficult to totally prevent the improper use of data stored in CPRs.

Because modern health care often requires shared care instead of care by a single physician only, the individual physician is no longer capable of personally guaranteeing the privacy of a patient's data. For that reason, after implementing regulations related to ensure the secrecy of patient data, modern societies must ensure the right to privacy. This means that in the different countries written regulations related to requests for personal data, including patient data, are required. These regulations should be supervised by a privacy committee and should contain descriptions of the purpose of the data registration that is maintained. It also should describe when data can be provided to third parties, and the right of all persons concerned to inspect, alter, and destroy their own data. In principle, these regulations do not concern data that have been made anonymous.

It is of utmost importance that in all (future) CPR systems proper measures be taken to protect the privacy of patients and their data. This issue is also the subject of discussions at the EU level, for example, in the standardization committees established for health care informatics and telematics. Some of the standardization activities related to CPRs are summarized in the following section.

Standardization

As discussed above, it is essential that standards for the acquisition, storage, and exchange of patient data be available. In health care this pertains to both administrative data and patient data. On the basis of the experiences over the past decade, a technical committee (TC 251 [De Moor and van Maele, 1996]) falling under CEN (*Comité Europeén de Normalisation,* the "European Committee for Standardization") was established. This committee defines preliminary standards and compiles reports on the standards to be introduced in the different countries of the European Union (De Moor, 1993; De Moor and van Maele, 1996). For instance, the ability to link systems via standard interfaces is widely recognized as a necessity. Especially in Europe, where data cross regional and national boundaries, agreement on how to exchange patient data is urgent. Directly and indirectly, such standards will contribute to the quality and efficiency of patient care.

From the long list of preliminary standards that have been or are being elaborated by Technical Committee 251, a few examples specifically dealing with data in CPRs are provided in the following sections (De Moor, 1996).

Electronic Health Care Record Architecture

Work on defining the basic architecture for data contained in an electronic health care record has begun. Standardization is necessary if patient data are to be exchanged between different health care professionals. It is also necessary so that patients can travel or move from one region or country in Europe to another. The architecture should enable physicians to use CPRs that are adapted to their own requirements and should therefore support a variety of formats. The aim of this standardization effort is not to specify the CPR system as such but to bring structure to the data stored in such records.

Coding Systems for Drugs

Standardization of coding systems for drugs concerns prescribing drugs and the effects of drugs on patients. A conceptual model for the correct labeling of drugs is foreseen within Technical Committee 251. The standard covers the identification of generic drug products as well as the drugs themselves. A coding system itself, however, is not intended.

Syntax for Health Care Data Interchange

Electronic messages in health care can be coded in many different ways. Therefore, consensus is required on the exchange formats for health care data between different systems. This has many advantages, because the systems' vendors can then handle the different data formats. The standard intends to define and adopt syntaxes for this exchange of information.

Exchange of Medical Images and Related Data

The medical image exchange standard concerns the exchange of high-volume data such as images or similar data. The Technical Committee 251 standard has adopted the industrial DICOM[6] 3.0 standard for medical images, enabling the possibility of standardized storage and global exchange of such images, which is important for supporting, for example, teleradiology or similar services.

User Identification

As open systems are gradually installed in hospitals and regional networks become operational, it will be important to prevent patient data from being used illegally. To ensure the proper use of patient data, it is necessary to positively identify authorized users. Software systems should therefore make use of automatic procedures for user identification, for example, by the use of passwords and different technical measures. Smart cards are other means of positive user identification (e.g., fingerprints or face recognition are possible techniques that could be standardized and that may eventually replace the more vulnerable passwords).

---

[6]DICOM: Digital Imaging and Communications standard (ACR-NEMA, 1985).

CONCLUSION

Significant progress has been made in Europe toward the primary recommendation of the IOM Committee on Improving the Patient Record's report over the past 6 years. Several factors account for the success to date. First, in those countries where CPRs are most prevalent, the health care delivery system or structure relies on a gatekeeper model and emphasizes primary health care and the health of the population. Thus, there is a recognized need for individual and aggregate patient data and a willingness to invest at both macro- (i.e., government) and microlevels (i.e., a practitioner) to make such data available. Second, CPR development projects are ideal for the EU insofar as they offer benefits both within and across countries and collaboration in their development may well speed up visible success. The evidence of political support and support by the medical professional organizations for CPRs sends a strong message to system developers and users, as well as to the general public.

Third, the emerging focus on conceptual models that build upon rather than are driven by the technology is a significant breakthrough in CPR development and will likely result in systems that can be adopted throughout Europe. Ultimately, this conceptual focus, which is also evident in the United States, may increase the ability of generic CPR systems to be transported globally. Fourth, collaboration between end-users and developers in system specification is a critical element of a sound CPR development process, aiding both the developers and users of the systems. Finally, the readiness of users with realistic expectations eases the implementation and increases the likelihood that CPRs will be used to their full potential. Thus, the education of health professionals is an important strategy in speeding CPR diffusion.

Like in the United States, important challenges remain to be addressed for CPR developers. First, continued support of CPR development efforts by supraregional and national organizations is absolutely essential. Second, the issues surrounding the operational exchange of patient data must be fully explored and addressed. Third, protecting the confidentiality of patient data in the information age is a global issue that must be a priority in all countries and will ultimately require greater collaboration among countries as the technologies that support CPRs continue to evolve and are exploited in ways that we have not yet identified. Fourth, flexible, user-adaptable generic models for the generation of CPRs are needed to overcome the great variety in specialized care, the differences in culture among various clinics, and particularly in Europe, among countries.

REFERENCES

ACR-NEMA (American College of Radiology and National Electrical Manufacturers Association). 1985. *Digital Imaging and Communications Standard 300-1985.* Washington, D.C.: NEMA Standards Publications.

Baud, R.H., A.M. Rassinoux, and J.-R. Scherrer. 1992. Natural language processing and semantical representation of medical texts. *Methods of Information in Medicine* 31(2):117-125.

Bakker, A. R. 1984. The development of an integrated and cooperative hospital information system. *Medical Informatics* 9:135-142.

Barber, B., A. Treacher, and K. Louwerse. 1996. *Toward Security in Medical Telematics. Studies in Health Technology and Informatics, No. 27*. Amsterdam: IOS Press.

Bernstein, K., and H. B. Jensen. 1994. Managing change in developing communication systems for integrated care; the Funen model. Pp. 266-269 in *Proceedings of Medical Informatics Europe 1994*, eds. P. Barahona, M. Veloso, and J. Bryant. Lisbon: Medical Informatics Europe.

Branger, P. J., J. C. van der Wouden, B. R. Schudel, E. Verboog, J. S. Duisterhout, J. van der Lei, and J. H. van Bemmel. 1992. Electronic communication between providers of primary and secondary care. *British Medical Journal* 305:1068-1070.

Branger, P. J., A. van't Hooft, J. S. Duisterhout, and J. van der Lei. 1994. A standardized message for supporting shared care. Pp. 473-477 in *Proceedings of the 18th Annual Symposium for Computer Applications in Medical Care*, ed. J. G. Ozbolt. (Special issue of the *Journal of the American Medical Informatics Association* 1994:473-477.)

Branger, P. J., and J .S. Duisterhout. 1995. Communication in health care. *Methods of Information in Medicine* 34:244-252.

Classen, D. C., S. L. Pestotnik, R. S. Evans, and J. P. Burke. 1991. Computerized surveillance of adverse drug events in hospital patients. *Journal of the American Medical Association* 266:2847-2851.

Degoulet, P., J. Coignard, F. C. Jean, et al. 1991. The Helios European project on software engineering. Pp. 125-137 in *Software Engineering in Medical Informatics*, eds. T. Timmers and B. I. Blum. Amsterdam: Elsevier Science.

De Moor, G. J. E. 1993. Standardization in medical informatics. Pp. 61-66 in *1993 Yearbook of Medical Informatics*, eds. J. H. van Bemmel and A. T. McCray. Stuttgart: Schattauer Verlag.

De Moor, G. J. E., and G. van Maele, eds. 1996. *Standards in Healthcare Informatics and Telematics*. Brussels: CEN/TC 251.

EU (European Union). 1994. *European Union DG XIII Work Programme on Health Telematics*. Brussels: Commission of the European Communities.

EU. 1995. European Union Directive 95/46/EC of the European Parliament and of the Council of 24 October 1995 "On the Protection of Individuals with Regard to the Processing of Personal Data and on the Free Movement of such Data." *Journal of the European Communities* 38:L281/31-50.

ISO (International Standards Organization). 1987. Electronic Data Interchange for Administration, Commerce and Transport (EDIFACT), Application Level Syntax Rules, IS 9735.

Kuilboer, M. M., and J. van der Lei. 1997. Exploring the role of a critiquing system: A simulation. *Journal of the American Medical Association* in press.

Lagouarde, P., R. Thomson, J.-L. Renaud-Salis, et al. 1996. The PROMPT electronic health care record. In *Proceedings of Medical Informatics in Europe 1996*, ed. P. McNair. Amsterdam: IOS Press.

Lamberts, H., and M. Wood, eds. 1987. *International Classification of Primary Care*. Oxford, England: Oxford University Press.

Millman, A., N. Lee, and A. Brooke. 1995. Computers in General Practice. Parts I, II, and III. *British Medical Journal* 311:800-802, 864-867, and 938-941.

Moorman, P. W., A. M. van Ginneken, J. van der Lei, and J. H. van Bemmel. 1994. A model for structured data entry based on explicit descriptional knowledge. *Methods of Information in Medicine* 33(5):454-463.

Nowlan, W.A, and A.L. Rector. 1991. Medical knowledge representation and predictive data entry. Pp. 105-116 in *Proceedings of Symposium on Artificial Intelligence in Medicine Europe*, ed. M. Stefanelli. Heidelberg: Springer-Verlag.

Nowlan, W. A., A. L. Rector, T. W. Rush, and W. D. Solomon. 1994. From terminology to terminology servers. Pp. 150-154 in *Proceedings of the 18th Annual Symposium for Computer Applications in Medical Care*, ed. J. G. Ozbolt. (Special issue of the Journal of the American Medical Informatics Association 1994:150-154.)

Nygren A., and P. Henriksson. 1992. Reading the medical record. I. Analysis of physicians' ways of reading the medical record. *Computer Methods and Programs in Biomedicine* 39:1-12.

OMG. 1996. *The Common Object Request Broker: Architecture and Specification* (V2.0). X/Open Publ.

Schaefer, O. P., and J. Sembritzki. 1996. German patient cards and the impact on interoperability. Pp. 137-139 in *Proceedings Toward an Electronic Patient Record '96,* ed. P. Waegemann. Newton, Mass.: Medical Records Institute.

Scherrer, J.-R., C. Louis, and F. Borst. 1995. Diogene 2, a distributed hospital information system with an emphasis on its medical information content. Pp. 86-97 in *1995 IMIA Yearbook of Medical Informatics,* eds. J. H. van Bemmel and A. T. McCray. Stuttgart: Schattauer Verlag.

Thomson, R. 1995. DILEMMA, decision support in primary are, oncology and shared care. Pp. 208-217 in *Health in the New Communication Age,* eds. M. F. Laires, M. J. Ladeira, and J. P. Christensen. Amsterdam: IOS Press.

Treaty for the Protection of Human Rights and Fundamental Freedom. Rome, 1954.

van Bemmel, J. H. 1992. Protection of medical data. Pp. 51-59 in *Cryptography and Data Protection. Proceedings of the Royal Netherlands Academy of Arts and Sciences, Vol. 38,* eds. J. H. van Lint and R. Tijdeman. Amsterdam: North-Holland.

van Bemmel, J. H. 1993. Criteria for the acceptance of decision-support systems by clinicians— lessons from ECG interpretation systems. Pp. 7-10 in *Proceedings of Symposium on Artificial Intelligence in Medicine Europe,* eds. S. Andreassen and J. Wyatt. Amsterdam: IOS Press.

van Bemmel, J. H., J. Fox, and K. Bernstein. 1996. Multimedia shared patient records—European experiences. Pp. 164-168 in *Proceedings Toward an Electronic Patient Record '96,* ed. P. Waegemann. Newton, Mass.: Medical Records Institute.

van der Lei, J., M. A. Musen, E. van der Does, A. Man in 't Veld, and J. H. van Bemmel. 1991a. Review of physician decision making using data from computer-stored medical records. *Lancet* 338:1504-1508.

van der Lei, J., and M. A. Musen. 1991b. A model for critiquing based on automated medical records. *Computers and Biomedical Research* 24:344-378.

van der Lei, J., J. S. Duisterhout, H. Westerhof, W. Boon, P. V. M. Cromme, and J. H. van Bemmel. 1993. The introduction of computer-based patient records in the Netherlands. *Annals of Internal Medicine* 119:1036-1041.

van Ginneken, A. M., J. van der Lei, and P. W. Moorman. 1993. Toward unambiguous representation of patient data. Pp. 69-73 in *Sixteenth Annual Symposium on Computer Applications in Medical Care,* ed. M. E. Frisse. New York: McGraw-Hill.

van Ginneken, A. M., H. Stam, and P. W. Moorman. 1995. A multi-strategy approach for medical records of specialists. Pp. 290-294 in *Proceedings of MEDINFO 95,* eds. R. A. Greenes, H. E. Peterson, and D. J. Protti. Vancouver, B.C.: Coach Publishing.

van Ginneken, A. M., and H. Stam. 1995. Can one patient record accommodate the diversity of specialized care? Pp. 406-410 in *Proceedings of the 19th Symposium on Computer Applications in Medical Care,* ed. R. M. Gardner. Philadelphia: Hanley & Belfus.

van Ginneken, A. M. 1996. Structured data entry: ORCA combines the strength of two models. In *Proceedings of the 20th Symposium on Computer Applications in Medical Care.* Philadelphia: Hanley & Belfus.

van Mulligen, E. M., T. Timmers, J. Brand, et al. 1994. Hermes: A health care workstation integration architecture. *International Journal of Biomedical Computing* 34:267-275.

Visser, L. E., A. E. Vlug, J. van der Lei, and B. H. Ch. Stricker. 1996. Cough due to ace inhibitors: A case-control study using automated general practice data. *European Journal of Clinical Pharmacology* 49:439-444.

Vlug, A. E., and J. van der Lei. 1995. Postmarketing surveillance with computer-based patient records. Pp 327-330 in *Proceedings of the 8th World Congress on Medical Informatics, MEDINFO 95*, eds. R. A. Greenes, H. E. Peterson, and D. J. Protti. Vancouver, B.C.: Coach Publishing.

Westerhof, H. P., W. M. Boon, P. V. M. Cromme, and J. H. van Bemmel. 1987. ELIAS: Support of the Dutch general practitioner. Pp 1-10 in *Present Status of Computer Support in Ambulatory Care*, eds. P. L. Reichertz, R. Engelbrecht, and U. Picollo. New York: Springer-Verlag.

Whiting-O'Keefe, Q. E., D. W. Simborg, W. V. Epstein, and A. Warger. 1985. A computerized summary medical record system can provide more information than the standard medical record. *Journal of the American Medical Association* 254(9):1185-1192.

Willems, J. L., C. Abreu-Lima, P. Arnaud, J. H. van Bemmel, et al. 1991. The diagnostic performance of computer programs for the interpretation of electrocardiograms. *New England Journal of Medicine* 325:1767-1773.

Wyatt, J. C. 1994. Clinical data systems. Part 3: Development and evaluation. *Lancet* 344:1682-1688.

Summary

The patient record touches, in some way, virtually everyone associated with providing, receiving, or reimbursing health care services. This wide range of application and use has led to efforts to automate the collection, storage, and management of the data that constitute these records. But in spite of more than 30 years of exploratory work and millions of dollars in research and implementation of computer systems in health care provider institutions, patient records today are still predominantly paper records. This evident lack of diffusion of information management technologies in the health care sector has limited the tools available for effective decision making from the bedside all the way to the formulation of national health care policy. Given the importance of patient data to the activities of all portions of the health care spectrum, the Institute of Medicine (IOM) undertook a study to improve patient records, acting in response to expanding demands for information and for increased functional capacity of patient record systems, as well as the considerable recent technological advances that bring the benefits of computer-based patient records within reach.

As its first step, the IOM study committee examined why previous work had not resulted in widespread improvement of patient records and asked whether and how another effort might be successful. The committee identified five conditions in the current health care environment that increase the likelihood of success.

1. The uses of and legitimate demands for patient data are growing. Part of this growth can be attributed to increased concern about the content and value of clinical therapies and a recent intense focus on health services research.

2. More powerful, affordable technologies to support computer-based patient records are now available.

3. Increasingly, computers are being accepted as a tool for enhancing efficiency in virtually all facets of everyday life.

4. Demographic factors such as an aging population (which results in a growth in chronic diseases) and the continued mobility of Americans create greater pressures for patient records that can manage large amounts of information and are easily transferable among health care providers.

5. Pressures for reform in health care are growing, and automation of patient records is crucial to achievement of such reform.

The combination of these factors led the committee to conclude that computerization can help to improve patient records and that improved patient records and information management of health care data are essential elements of the infrastructure of the nation's health care system.

USER NEEDS AND SYSTEM REQUIREMENTS

The patient record of the future will have many more users and uses than it has at present. Direct providers of care (physicians, nurses, dentists, and other health care professionals) will remain the users of highest priority in design considerations. However, with the expanded functions projected for patient records (e.g., their use in supplying data for research or for insurance claims), the range of users considered in record system design will widen. The needs of all users will be met to an extent not possible in current record systems. Ultimately, of course, the most significant beneficiary of improved patient records should be the patient.

The committee identified five objectives for future patient record systems. First, future patient records should support patient care and improve its quality. Second, they should enhance the productivity of health care professionals and reduce the administrative costs associated with health care delivery and financing. Third, they should support clinical and health services research. Fourth, they should be able to accommodate future developments in health care technology, policy, management, and finance. Fifth, they must have mechanisms in place to ensure patient data confidentiality at all times.

To achieve these objectives, future patient records must be computer based. However, merely automating the form, content, and procedures of current patient records will perpetuate their deficiencies and will be insufficient to meet emerging user needs. The committee defined the computer-based patient record as an electronic patient record that resides in a system specifically designed to support users through availability of complete and accurate data, practitioner reminders and alerts, clinical decision support

systems, links to bodies of medical knowledge, and other aids. This definition encompasses a broader view of the patient record than is current today,
moving from the notion of a location or device for keeping track of patient
care events to a resource with much enhanced utility in patient care (including the ability to provide an accurate longitudinal account of care), in management of the health care system, and in extension of knowledge.

In the past, a patient record has served the basic function of storing
patient data for retrieval by users involved with providing patient care.
Even this classic function must be broader in the future, however, especially with respect to the key feature of flexibility. Different health care
professionals will require different modes of record information retrieval
and display. Today, both paper and computer records are often cumbersome tools for these tasks. The record of the future must be far more
flexible, allowing its users to design and utilize reporting formats tailored
to their own special needs and to organize and display data in various ways.

The patient record system of the future must provide other capabilities as
well, including links to administrative, bibliographic, clinical knowledge,
and research databases. To meet the needs of clinicians, CPR systems must
be linked to decision support systems; they must also support video or
picture graphics and must provide electronic mail capability within and
between provider settings.

Future CPR systems must offer enhanced communications capabilities to
meet emerging user needs. The systems must be able to transmit detailed
records reliably across substantial distances. Physician offices must be able
to communicate with local hospitals and national bibliographic resources.
In hospitals, all of the various departmental systems (e.g., finance, laboratory, nursing, radiology) must be able to communicate with the patient
record system. In the larger health care environment, computer-based information management systems must be able to communicate with providers, third-party payers, and other health care entities, while at all times
maintaining confidentiality of the information.

If users are to derive maximum benefits from future patient record systems, they must fulfill four conditions. First, users must have confidence in
the data—which implies that the individual who collects data must be able
to enter them directly into the system and that the system must be able to
reliably integrate data from all sources and accurately retrieve them whenever necessary. Second, they must use the record actively in the clinical
process. Third, they must understand that the record is a resource for use
beyond direct patient care—for example, to study the effectiveness and
efficiency of clinical processes, procedures, and technologies. Fourth, they
must be proficient in the use of future computer-based record systems (i.e.,
the systems described in this report) and the tools that such systems provide
(e.g., links to bibliographic databases or clinical decision support systems).

COMPUTER-BASED PATIENT RECORD TECHNOLOGIES

Over the past decades, progress has been steady toward developing complete CPR systems, and several powerful clinical information systems have become operational in recent years. Typically, development of these systems began at least a decade ago, and some have been under development for more than two decades. *No current system, however, is capable of supporting the complete CPR.*

Those clinical information systems that most closely approximate the CPR system envisioned by the committee share several common traits. First, they maintain a large data dictionary to define the contents of their internal CPRs. Second, all patient data recorded in the CPR are tagged with the time and date of the transaction, thus making the CPR a continuous chronological history of the patient's medical care. Third, the systems retrieve and report data in the CPR in a flexible manner. Finally, the systems offer a research tool for using the CPR data.

Most of the technological barriers that formerly impeded development of CPR systems have either disappeared already or are about to dissolve. Nevertheless, although no technological breakthroughs are needed to realize CPR systems, further maturation of a few emerging technologies, such as hand-held computers, voice-input or voice-recognition systems, and text-processing systems may be necessary to develop state-of-the-art CPR systems in the 1990s. In some cases, promising technologies must be tested further in "real-life" situations; in other cases, technologies that have proved beneficial in applications in other fields must be adopted for use in health care.

In addition to further development of necessary technologies, a variety of standards must be developed, tested, and implemented before the CPR can realize its full potential at both the macro (e.g., epidemiological) and micro (e.g., physician office) levels. Standards to facilitate the exchange of health care data are needed so that clinical data may be transmitted on networks or aggregated and analyzed to support improved decision making. Standards are also needed for the development of more secure CPR systems. This effort should focus on ensuring the integrity of the clinical data in the CPR and protecting its confidentiality. It is crucial that confidentiality be maintained in CPR systems not only for the patient but also for health care professionals.

NONTECHNOLOGICAL BARRIERS

In addition to technological advances, successful implementation of CPR systems requires elimination of the barriers to development (i.e., the production of new capabilities) and diffusion. It also requires that the concerns of many interested parties be addressed and that individuals and organizations with resources to support needed changes be engaged in the effort.

Many impediments to the CPR and to CPR systems arise from a lack of awareness and understanding of their capabilities and benefits. The intellectual understanding of what needs to be done, how to do it, and for whom to do it—that is, the demanding collection of insights required for design—is a continuing problem that must be addressed. (For example, when users are asked what capabilities they would like to have available to them, they may have difficulty imagining what CPR systems will be able to do in the future.) System purchasers and users often lack adequate information about the benefits and costs of the CPR. Developers and vendors require more specific information about what users want from systems and what price providers would be willing to pay for systems that meet their needs. Activities aimed at improving and disseminating available information about CPR systems—for instance, through demonstration projects and education programs—constitute an important step toward CPR implementation.

Other impediments arise from the lack of an infrastructure to support CPR development and diffusion. Needed infrastructure components are standards for communication of data (i.e., vocabulary control and data format standards); laws and regulations that protect patient privacy but do not inhibit transfer of information to legitimate users of data outside the clinical setting; experts trained in the development and use of CPR systems; institutional, local, regional, and national networks for transmitting CPR data; reimbursement mechanisms that pay for the costs of producing improved patient care information; and a management structure (i.e., an organization) for setting priorities, garnering and allocating resources, and coordinating activities.

Consideration of the various barriers to CPR development, the interest and resources of individuals and organizations able to effect change, and the concerns of individuals who would be affected by implementation of CPRs prompted the committee to identify eight critical activities that will help advance CPR development: (1) identification and understanding of CPR design requirements; (2) development of standards; (3) CPR and CPR systems research and development; (4) demonstrations of effectiveness, costs, and benefits of CPR systems; (5) reduction of legal constraints for CPR uses as well as enhancement of legal protection for patients; (6) coordination of resources and support for CPR development and diffusion; (7) coordination of information and resources for secondary patient record databases; and (8) education and training of developers and users.

Accomplishing these activities will require adequate funding and effective organization. The committee reviewed organizational structures that could provide the necessary framework for coordinating CPR activities and concluded that no existing organization has the mandate and resources necessary to lead the CPR effort. Thus, for reasons set forth more fully in Chapter 4, the committee believes that a new organization is needed to

BOX 1 SUMMARY OF THE RECOMMENDATIONS OF THE INSTITUTE OF MEDICINE COMMITTEE ON IMPROVING THE PATIENT RECORD

The committee recommends the following:

1. Health care professionals and organizations should adopt the computer-based patient record (CPR) as the standard for medical and all other records related to patient care.

2. To accomplish Recommendation No. 1, the public and private sectors should join in establishing a Computer-based Patient Record Institute (CPRI) to promote and facilitate development, implementation, and dissemination of the CPR.

3. Both the public and private sectors should expand support for the CPR and CPR system implementation through research, development, and demonstration projects. Specifically, the committee recommends that Congress authorize and appropriate funds to implement the research and development agenda outlined herein. The committee further recommends that private foundations and vendors fund programs that support and facilitate this research and development agenda.

4. The CPRI should promulgate uniform national standards for data and security to facilitate implementation of the CPR and its secondary databases.

5. The CPRI should review federal and state laws and regulations for the purpose of proposing and promulgating model legislation and regulations to facilitate the implementation and dissemination of the CPR and its secondary databases and to streamline the CPR and CPR systems.

6. The costs of CPR systems be should shared by those who benefit from the value of the CPR. Specifically, the full costs of implementing and operating CPRs and CPR systems should be factored into reimbursement levels or payment schedules of both public and private sector third-party payers. In addition, users of secondary databases should support the costs of creating such databases.

7. Health care professional schools and organizations should enhance educational programs for students and practitioners in the use of computers, CPRs, and CPR systems for patient care, education, and research.

support CPR development and implementation. The committee has proposed a framework for the establishment of such an organization, but it also emphasizes that achieving adequate resources for and engaging the appropriate parties in CPR development efforts are more important than the precise structure of the recommended organization.

RECOMMENDATIONS

The committee believes its recommendations (see Box 1) effectively address the potential barriers to routine CPR use. The first recommendation defines CPRs and CPR systems as the standard for future patient records; the second proposes an organizational framework within which barriers to CPR implementation can be systematically addressed and overcome. The remaining recommendations focus on specific impediments: needed research and development, promulgation of standards for CPR data and security, review of legal constraints and remedies, distribution of costs for CPR systems, and education of health care professionals.

The committee believes that the CPR can play an increasingly important role in the health care environment. This role begins in the care process as the CPR provides patient information when needed and supports clinical decision making. It extends to management of care through the establishment of a mechanism by which quality assurance procedures and clinical practice guidelines are accessible to health care professionals at the time and site of patient care. It also includes opportunities for reducing administrative costs and frustrations associated with health care financing and for capturing administrative data for internal and external review. Finally, the CPR's role extends to capturing relevant, accurate data necessary for provider and consumer education, technology assessment, health services research, and related work concerning the appropriateness, effectiveness, and outcomes of care.

The committee recognizes the considerable amount of work that remains to be done and the practical limitations that must be overcome before CPRs become the standard mode of documenting and communicating patient information and before they are perceived and used as a vital resource for improving patient care. The challenge of coordinating CPR development efforts in the pluralistic health care environment is great. Resources are limited and must be used wisely.

The committee is convinced that proper coordination and appropriate resources will lead to achievement of the goal of widespread CPR utilization within a decade. The desire to improve the quality of and access to patient data is shared by patients, practitioners, administrators, third-party payers, researchers, and policymakers throughout the nation. CPRs and CPR systems can respond to health care's need for a "central nervous system" to manage the complexities of modern medicine—from patient care to public health to health care policy. In short, the CPR is an essential technology for health care today and in the future.

1

Introduction

The patient record is the principal repository for information concerning a patient's health care. It affects, in some way, virtually everyone associated with providing, receiving, or reimbursing health care services. Despite the many technological advances in health care over the past few decades, the typical patient record of today is remarkably similar to the patient record of 50 years ago. This failure of patient records to evolve is now creating additional stress within the already burdened U.S. health care system as the information needs of practitioners,[1] patients, administrators, third-party payers, researchers, and policymakers often go unmet. As described by Ellwood (1988:1550),

> The intricate machinery of our health care system can no longer grasp the threads of experience. . . . Too often, payers, physicians, and health care executives do not share common insights into the life of the patient. . . . The health care system has become an organism guided by misguided choices; it is unstable, confused, and desperately in need of a central nervous system that can help it cope with the complexities of modern medicine.

Patient record improvement could make major contributions to improving the health care system of this nation. A 1991 General Accounting Office (GAO) report on automated medical records identified three major ways in which improved patient records could benefit health care (GAO,

---

[1]The committee uses the term *practitioners* to refer to all health care professionals who provide clinical services to patients. These professionals include, but are not limited to, physicians, nurses, dentists, and therapists.

1991). First, automated patient records can improve health care delivery by providing medical personnel with better data access, faster data retrieval, higher quality data, and more versatility in data display. Automated patient records can also support decision making and quality assurance activities and provide clinical reminders to assist in patient care. Second, automated patient records can enhance outcomes research programs by electronically capturing clinical information for evaluation. Third, automated patient records can increase hospital efficiency by reducing costs and improving staff productivity.

Several sources support these conclusions. The GAO reported that an automated medical record system reduced hospital costs by $600 per patient in a Department of Veterans Affairs hospital because of shorter hospital stays (GAO, 1991). Reductions in the length of inpatient stays were also found in other studies of computerized medical records and medical record summaries (Rogers and Haring, 1979). Other investigators found enhanced care and improved outcome of care for clinic patients (Rogers et al., 1982) and a reduction in medication errors (Garrett et al., 1986).

The first step toward patient record improvement is a close examination of the users of the patient record, the technologies available to create and maintain it, and the barriers to enhancing it. To that end, the Institute of Medicine (IOM) of the National Academy of Sciences undertook a study to recommend improvements to patient records in response to expanding functional requirements and technological advances.[2] This report is the product of the multidisciplinary panel's 18-month study of how patient records can be improved to meet the many and varied demands for patient information and to enhance the quality of patient care and the effectiveness and efficiency of health care delivery.

THE STUDY

The idea for this study originated in discussions between staff at the National Institutes of Health (NIH) and IOM. The NIH staff were involved in patient care, teaching, and research and were motivated by the need to make patient records more useful for all of these purposes. The IOM

---

[2]The IOM committee was originally named the Committee on Improving the Medical Record in Response to Increasing Functional Requirements and Technological Advances. The committee's first action was to change "medical" to "patient" in its name, reflecting its consensus that the medical component of the record does not constitute the total record. Thus, this report generally will refer to what are commonly called medical records as "patient records." There are several instances, however, in which the committee continues to refer to medical records rather than patient records. For example, the committee's official charge relates to medical records, and the committee has not undertaken to rename "medical record professionals."

was considered to be an ideal agent to bring together the diverse perspectives needed to address a broad range of patient record issues. Thus, the participants at a June 1986 IOM program development workshop recommended that the institute conduct a study of the patient record in light of new technologies. Subsequently, staff of the IOM Council on Health Care Technology developed an action plan for the study, which was approved by the National Research Council in July 1987. Efforts to enlist adequate financial support occurred over the ensuing two years.

The IOM appointed a study committee in March 1989, and the committee began its deliberations the following September. Among its membership were experts in community and academic medicine, health information services, health services research, hospital services, medical information systems, regulatory functions, and third-party payment.

The Committee's Charge

In general, the IOM study committee was charged to examine the problems with existing medical record systems and to propose actions and research for their improvement in light of new technologies. Specifically, the committee was asked to:

• examine the current state of medical record systems, including their availability, use, strengths, and weaknesses;
• identify impediments to the development and use of improved record systems;
• identify ways, including developments now in progress, to overcome impediments and improve medical record systems;
• develop a research agenda to advance medical record systems;
• develop a plan, design, and/or other provisions for improved medical record systems, including a means for updating these systems and the research agenda as appropriate; and
• recommend policies and other strategies to achieve these improvements.

In addition to addressing the technological issues in its charge, the committee sought to produce a report that would increase the interest of all health care practitioners in improving patient records and health care information management. Involvement of these practitioners in the development of future patient records is required if record improvement efforts are to meet with success.

Committee Activities

The committee met five times between September 1989 and December 1990. It established three subcommittees—Users and Uses, Technology, and Strategy and Implementation (see Appendix A). The subcommittees, each with approximately 15 members, met at least twice and solicited information from more than 70 advisers, including physicians (in both private practice and academic medicine), nurses, dentists, medical record professionals, hospital administrators, researchers, and congressional staff. Also among these advisers were representatives of patient groups, computer software and hardware vendors, third-party payers, government agencies, and professional organizations. Each subcommittee prepared a report that was considered, along with the results of a special workshop and several background papers, by the full committee in its deliberations.

Definitions

During its work, the committee used the following specific definitions:

• A *patient record* is the repository of information about a single patient. This information is generated by health care professionals as a direct result of interaction with a patient or with individuals who have personal knowledge of the patient (or with both). Traditionally, patient records have been paper and have been used to store patient care data.

• A *computer-based patient record* (CPR) is an electronic patient record that resides in a system specifically designed to support users by providing accessibility to complete and accurate data, alerts, reminders, clinical decision support systems,[3] links to medical knowledge, and other aids.

• A *primary patient record* is used by health care professionals while providing patient care services to review patient data or document their own observations, actions, or instructions.

• A *secondary patient record* is derived from the primary record and contains selected data elements to aid nonclinical users (i.e., persons not involved in direct patient care) in supporting, evaluating, or advancing patient care.[4] Patient care support refers to administration, regulation, and

---

[3]Shortliffe and colleagues define a clinical decision support system as "any computer system designed to help health professionals make clinical decisions" (Shortliffe et al., 1990:469). They identify three types of decision support functions: information management, focusing of attention, and patient-specific consultation. Throughout this report, *clinical decision support systems* refer to clinical consultation systems that use population statistics or encode expert knowledge to assist practitioners in diagnosis or in formulating treatment plans (Shortliffe et al., 1990).

[4]The committee's distinction between primary and secondary patient records parallels, but is not identical to, the approach used by Westin (1976). Westin identified three "zones" through which information flows: (1) direct patient care, (2) supporting activities, and (3) social uses of health data. This report does not address social uses of patient care data that lie outside health care (e.g., law enforcement) and combines supporting activities and health care social uses of patient data into one zone.

payment functions. Patient care evaluation refers to quality assurance, utilization review, and medical or legal audits. Patient care advancement refers to research. These records are often combined to form what the committee terms a secondary database (e.g., an insurance claims database).

• A *patient record system* is the set of components that form the mechanism by which patient records are created, used, stored, and retrieved. A patient record system is usually located within a health care provider setting. It includes people, data, rules and procedures, processing and storage devices (e.g., paper and pen, hardware and software), and communication and support facilities.

A patient record system can be part of a *hospital information system,* which typically handles both administrative and clinical functions, or a *medical information system,* which has been defined as "the set of formal arrangements by which the facts concerning the health or health care of individual patients are stored and processed in computers" (Lindberg, 1979:9). A patient record system is a type of *clinical information system,* which is dedicated to collecting, storing, manipulating, and making available clinical information important to the delivery of patient care. The central focus of such systems is clinical data and not financial or billing information. Such systems may be limited in their scope to a single area of clinical information (e.g., dedicated to laboratory data), or they may be comprehensive and cover virtually every facet of clinical information pertinent to patient care (e.g., computer-based patient record systems).

REPORT ORGANIZATION

The remainder of this chapter discusses the current state of patient record systems, including their strengths and weaknesses, and the environment of opportunity that exists for implementing computer-based patient records. Chapter 2 delineates the needs of patient record users and describes how future patient record systems can meet user needs. Chapter 3 identifies technologies essential to future systems and assesses how well existing systems meet future requirements. Chapter 4 describes nontechnological barriers to improving patient records and presents a strategic plan for overcoming them. Finally, Chapter 5 sets forth the committee's recommendations for accelerating the realization of computer-based patient records and suggests an agenda for their implementation and dissemination within a decade.

THE PATIENT RECORD

Virtually every person in the United States who has received health care since 1918 has a patient record (MacEachern, 1937). Today, most people have multiple patient records—one for each health care provider they have visited. Patient records have proliferated to the extent that some medical centers in large metropolitan areas may now each have more than 4 million paper patient records (Kurland and Molgaard, 1981). Although at any one time these records are not all active, they must be stored for up to 25 years, depending on state laws (Waller, in this volume). Moreover, a given patient may have more than one record even within a particular institution.[5]

Patient records appear in a variety of forms—for example, as paper; microfilm; a monitor strip; an optical disk; a computer card, tape, or disk; or a combination of these (Amatayakul and Wogan, 1989). They are created and used most frequently in health care provider settings such as physician or dentist offices, hospitals, nursing homes, and public health clinics; but other institutions such as correctional institutions, the armed forces, occupational health programs of employers, and colleges and universities also maintain patient health care records (Westin, 1976).[6]

For more than a century, the paper patient record has been the primary vehicle for recording patient care information (Huffman, 1981). Yet recent years have seen a trend toward automation of components of patient records (e.g., clinical laboratory test results) or certain patient care functions (e.g., entering physician orders for hospitalized patients; Westin, 1976; Gardner and Perry, 1989; Amatayakul and Sattler, 1990). Some hospitals, health maintenance organizations, and physicians' offices now have prototype elements of computer-based record systems.[7] These facilities are still the exception rather than the rule, however, and paper patient records, with their sometimes overlooked strengths and frequently cited weaknesses, are still the norm for most health care providers.

Strengths and Weaknesses of Paper Patient Records

The committee's literature review did not reveal any substantive documentation of the strengths of paper patient records. This result may be

---

[5]Health care professionals might maintain a separate patient record to protect sensitive data (e.g., psychiatric history) or to support a research interest (i.e., separate records containing detailed data for a research project).

[6]Pharmacies capture information pertinent to patient care but do not maintain full patient records. Information on the medications prescribed and the specialties of the physicians writing the prescriptions can provide enough information to determine a patient's medical problems, however, and pharmacy records may thus raise confidentiality issues similar to those associated with patient records. Because the committee focused more closely on traditional patient care records, this report does not address issues related to pharmacy records.

[7]Chapter 3 highlights some of the health care provider institutions at the leading edge of patient record technologies.

explained in part by the facts that the value of maintaining patient records is widely accepted in the health care community and that paper is the most widely used record-keeping form. Given the prevalence of paper patient records, the committee noted that support by practitioners for this kind of record keeping should not be underestimated. Time and resource constraints did not permit the committee to survey user attitudes toward paper records; however, committee members identified at least five strengths of such records from the perspective of record users:

1. Paper records are familiar to users who consequently do not need to acquire new skills or behaviors to use them.

2. Paper records are portable and can be carried to the point of care.

3. Once in hand, paper records do not experience downtime as computer systems do.

4. Paper records allow flexibility in recording data and are able to record "soft" (i.e., subjective) data easily.[8]

5. Paper records can be browsed through and scanned (if they are not too large). This feature allows users to organize data in various ways and to look for patterns or trends that are not explicitly stated.

Criticism of current patient records is sometimes sharp. Burnum (1989:484) states that "[m]edical records, which have long been faulty, contain more distorted, deleted, and misleading information than ever before." Pories (1990:47) relates the story of an engineer who was asked to recommend more efficient use of health care personnel but who instead was "stunned by the disorganization of the medical record and the inefficiencies it imposed on the delivery of care." The engineer concluded that "the redesign of the record offered the most immediate and simple approach for medical cost control and for prevention of malpractice" (p. 47).

Pories believes that this situation has not improved and that it is not isolated. "No one has a monopoly on the problem: medical records appear to be equally bad and dangerous throughout the land" (Pories, 1990:47). He is not alone in his view that patient records often lack the features needed for their most beneficial use. In a recent survey of internists in academic and private practice, 63 percent of the respondents agreed with the statement that patient records are becoming increasingly burdensome without improving the quality of patient care (Hershey et al., 1989).

The weaknesses of patient records, as described in the literature and in the work of the committee, can be subsumed under four main headings: (1)

---

[8]Although flexibility in recording data may be viewed as a strength by the individual recording the information, lack of standard vocabulary and coding can pose problems for subsequent users—including practitioners, administrators, researchers, and third-party payers.

content; (2) format; (3) access, availability, and retrieval; and (4) linkages and integration.

Problems with Patient Record Content

Patient record data are often missing, illegible, or inaccurate (Tufo and Speidel, 1971; Zuckerman et al., 1975; Bentsen, 1976; Zimmerman, 1978; Fox et al., 1979; Romm and Putnam, 1981; Gerbert and Hargreaves, 1986; Hsia et al., 1988; Pories, 1990). Data can be missing for at least three reasons: (1) questions were never asked, examinations were never performed, or tests were never ordered; (2) the information was requested and provided, but either it was not recorded by the clinician or delays occurred in placing the information in the record; and (3) the information was requested and delivered but was misplaced or lost. In addition, clinicians, patients, or equipment can all introduce errors into patient records (Burnum, 1989).

Many studies have examined the quality of patient record content. Table 1-1 presents the findings of several such investigations. The missing information reported in the various studies often resulted in additional costs of patient care. For example, an estimated 11 percent of laboratory tests in one hospital were ordered to duplicate tests for which findings were unavailable to the physician at the time of the patient visit (Tufo and Speidel, 1971).

Although for some records data are missing, in other cases certain data are excessive or redundant (Zimmerman, 1978; Korpman and Lincoln, 1988). The thickness and weight of the records of patients with chronic problems can be imposing, if not daunting, and time constraints may prevent the user from finding and using necessary information. (In one study of paper patient records, the average weight of a clinic record was 1-1/2 pounds [Rogers et al., 1982].) Other issues related to record content include failure to capture the rationale of providers, lack of standardization of definitions of terminology, failure to describe the patient experience, lack of patient-based generic health outcome measures, and incomprehensibility for patients and their families.

Problems with Format

Several studies have pointed to patient record formats as a problem area that at times impedes record use and effectiveness. The 1980 IOM study cited in Table 1-1 found that the reliability of hospital discharge data depended on the general organization, orderliness, and logic of the medical record. Zimmerman (1978) conducted a survey of physicians who identified poor organization of medical records as a deficiency that contributed

TABLE 1-1 Selected Parameters and Findings of Studies of Patient Record Content

Author(s)/Parameters	Study Data
Tufo and Speidel (1971)	
Purpose	Evaluate record availability, missing data, recording of laboratory results, incomplete physician narrative, and data collected for general health evaluations
Sample	1,149 patient visits in five outpatient U.S. Army facilities
Findings	11% of patients had no past medical data available
	5-20% of charts had information missing:
	75% of missing data were laboratory test results or reports of radiologic examinations
	25% of missing data were lost, incomplete, or illegible data from previous visits
	13-79% of laboratory results were not placed in the record
	10-49% of visits did not have a well-defined problem in the record
	6-49% of visits did not have a well-defined treatment in the record
	40-73% of records did not have evidence of general medical information useful for preventive medicine
Dawes (1972)	
Purpose	Determine presence of 18 data elements
Sample	1,628 medical records (the last episode of disease) in general practices
Findings	10% of patient ages were not recorded
	30% of episodes had no therapeutic agent recorded; of those recorded, 75% were missing the amount prescribed, and 80% were missing dosages
	40% of episodes had no diagnosis recorded
	60% of males and 77% of females had no occupation recorded
	99% of males and 21% of females had no marital status recorded
Zuckerman et al. (1975)	
Purpose	Appraise the extent to which records document adequately the content of verbal communication between physicians and patients
Sample	51 tape-recorded physician-patient encounters in pediatric clinic
Findings	Percent present on tape and absent on record:
	0% of chief complaints
	6% of reason for visit
	10% of degree of disability
	12% of allergies
	22% of compliance data
	31% of indications for follow-up
	51% of cause of illness
Bentsen (1976)	
Purpose	Assess the validity of data in the information system of the department
Sample	59 patient encounters in family medicine clinics
Findings	41% of problems identified by observers were not recorded

TABLE 1-1 (Continued)

Author(s)/Parameters	Study Data
IOM (1980)	
Purpose	Assess the reliability of data collected as part of the National Hospital Discharge Survey
Sample	3,313 medical records from 66 hospitals that participated in the National Hospital Discharge Survey
Findings	75% of face sheets had no discharge disposition
	48% of face sheets were inadequate for determining principal diagnosis
	15% of face sheets and discharge summaries were inadequate for determining principal diagnosis
Romm and Putnam (1981)	
Purpose	Document extent of agreement between the record and the verbal content of the physician-patient encounter
Sample	55 patient encounters in general medicine clinics
Findings	Percent agreement between record and observation of encounter:
	29% for other medical history
	66% for therapy
	71% for information related to current illness
	72% for tests
	73% for impression/diagnosis
	92% for chief complaint
Hsia et al. (1988)	
Purpose	Verify coding of diagnosis-related groups (DRGs)
Sample	7,050 medical records of Medicare patients from 239 hospitals
Findings	20.8% of the discharges were coded incorrectly (in the direction of higher weighted DRGs)

to ineffective use. The format of the usual paper record does not lend itself easily to dealing with multiple problems over a long period of time. For example, Pories (1990) noted that the physical form of paper records (i.e., binders or charts) is often unmanageable; data are fragmented within the record and not sorted for relevance. Fries (1974) showed that information could be found four times faster in a structured flow sheet than in a traditional paper medical record and that 10 percent of items in the traditional record could not be found.

Traditionally, patient records are organized according to the sources and chronology of data (Feinstein, 1970), although several alternative record formats have been developed. For example, the problem-oriented medical record (POMR) is assembled according to the patient's problems to support a more organized approach to clinical problem solving and management

(Weed, 1968). The summary time-oriented record (STOR) is an outpatient medical record system that consists of a concise summary of a patient's clinical data that can be used either in conjunction with the traditional medical record or by itself (Whiting-O'Keefe et al., 1985).

Problems with Access, Availability, and Retrieval

Record unavailability and difficulties in accessing records when they are available are frequent problems for patient record users (Pories, 1990). Tufo and Speidel (1971) documented in their study that medical records were unavailable in up to 30 percent of patient visits. They attributed this rate of unavailability to several possible causes: patients being seen in two or more clinics on the same day, charts not being forwarded, physicians keeping records in their offices or removing them from their offices, and records being misfiled in the file room. One hospital in the GAO study on automated medical records reported that it could not locate medical records 30 percent of the time (GAO, 1991). Even when records are readily available, the amount of time required to retrieve necessary information from a record can frustrate users (Fries, 1974; Zimmerman, 1978; Pories, 1990).

For researchers, access to paper records can be problematic and is generally resource intensive (Davies, 1990). Identifying records that contain needed data, retrieving needed records, reviewing records, collecting data, and entering data into data sets for analysis are time-consuming, expensive tasks. Yet access to existing computer-based records can also prove difficult for researchers because documentation on how to use systems may be lacking. Further, data aggregation can be hampered by lack of compatibility among systems.

Problems with Linkages and Integration

One of the major criticisms of the U.S. health care system is the discontinuity of care among providers (Rulin et al., 1988; Case and Jones, 1989). This discontinuity extends to patient records, whose lack of integration of inpatient and outpatient information is a significant deficiency. Paper patient records offer little hope of improving the coordination of health care services within or among provider institutions. Moreover, the inadequacy of patient record interfaces with other clinical data, administrative information, or medical knowledge impedes optimal use of record information in providing patient care. Several health care systems and institutions have developed records that overcome many of the problems associated with traditional paper records, but even these improved records suffer from their lack of easy transferability to other health care provider systems or institutions.

Outpatient Records

Attention is frequently focused on patient records in hospitals rather than in outpatient settings. (An inpatient record is used by many different individuals during an episode of illness, so its weaknesses can appear quite pronounced.) Yet outpatient records are greater in number, are scattered among individual physician offices, and may exhibit even greater variance in quality than inpatient records. There are no established standards or review organizations for outpatient records as there are for inpatient records. As a result, outpatient records often serve as files for "correspondence and reports rather than as a well organized chronology of health care" (Pories, 1990:49).

Ambulatory care records frequently contain poorly organized data, lack documentation of key aspects of care, and exhibit inaccurate diagnostic coding (IOM, 1990c). Health care researchers and clinicians who conduct retrospective studies using such records are likely to identify at least four weaknesses: lack of standardization in content and format, inaccessibility (except in some hospitals or large health plans), incompleteness, and inaccuracies (Davies, 1990).

INFORMATION MANAGEMENT CHALLENGES

An Information-Intensive Industry

Providing high-quality health care services is an information-dependent process. Indeed, the practice of medicine has been described as being "dominated" by how well information is processed or reprocessed, retrieved, and communicated (Barnett, 1990). An estimated 35 to 39 percent of total hospital operating costs have been associated with patient and professional communication activities (Richart, 1970). Physicians spend an estimated 38 percent (Mamlin and Baker, 1973) and nurses an estimated 50 percent (Korpman and Lincoln, 1988) of their time writing up patient charts.

Information-processing activities associated with providing health services to patients are extremely varied. Clinicians obtain and record information about patients, consult with colleagues, read scientific literature, select diagnostic procedures, interpret results of laboratory studies, devise strategies for patient care, instruct allied health professionals, discuss care plans with patients and families, and document the progress of patients. In addition, health care practitioners must distill knowledge, interpret data, apply knowledge, and manage the complexities of medical decision making (Haynes et al., 1989; Greenes and Shortliffe, 1990). Thus, health care professionals routinely need access to appropriate compilations of thorough, up-to-date knowledge and advice to make prompt, informed decisions regarding patient care (Haynes et al., 1989; Saba et al., 1989; Greenes and Shortliffe, 1990). Furthermore, a wide range of information-processing tasks supports patient care, including performing laboratory tests, processing medical imaging data, capturing patient demographic information, filling prescription orders, monitoring quality and appropriateness of services provided, and billing (Martin, 1990).

An Information Explosion

For the past several years, health care practitioners have faced an explosion in medical knowledge. For instance, MEDLINE[9] now indexes approximately 360,000 new articles each year from those published in the biomedical literature (National Institutes of Health, 1989). Scientific and technological advances that have contributed to improving the health of the public have also resulted in more complexity in medical practice; clinicians must track ever more numerous diagnoses, procedures, diagnostic tests, clinical processes, devices, and drugs.

The increase in available technologies places an additional burden on physicians: they must read and synthesize the literature and try to decide whether and how new technologies should be applied (Brook, 1989). Often, a gap occurs between the information physicians need and the information available to them at the time of providing patient care. According to Covell and colleagues (1985), an estimated 70 percent of physician information needs are unmet during the patient visit.

In addition to more knowledge, there are more data for health care professionals to manage. The volume and complexity of information per patient have increased owing to a greater number of patient encounters (as patients live longer and experience chronic disease), higher patient acuity of illness (both in and out of hospitals), more kinds of clinical data elements arising from new diagnostic technologies, and developments in the delivery system that result in many patients receiving care at multiple sites. Concomitant with increases in information, however, have been efforts to reduce unit costs of health care provider institutions, which create pressures on health care professionals to be more productive and to see more patients. This paradoxically reduces the time and energy available for the functions associated with management and communication of information. Health care professionals are thus placed in a frustrating, difficult, and perhaps untenable position.

---

[9]MEDLINE is an on-line bibliographic database of medical information. It covers 25 years and includes citations to more than 6 million articles from approximately 3,500 journals. MEDLINE is part of the National Library of Medicine Medical Literature Analysis and Retrieval System (MEDLARS), which includes specialized databases in health administration, toxicology, cancer, medical ethics, and population studies (National Institutes of Health, 1989).

Increasing Demand for Data

Even as patient care data become more voluminous and complex, the demand by multiple users for access to patient care data is increasing (Barnett, 1990). Information must be shared among the multiplicity of health care professionals who constitute the "health care team." These professionals represent the physician specialties, as well as nurses, dentists, therapists, pharmacists, technicians, social workers, and other health care providers. Patients may also require access to records; some providers advocate greater patient input into the process of care through patient identification of preferences among treatments, patient contributions to the record (particularly history and functional status; Davies and Ware, 1988; Donnelly, 1988; Tarlov et al., 1989), patient reading and validation of record data, and patient control and transport of pertinent parts of the record (Tufo et al., 1977; Bronson et al., 1978).

Administrators and managers of health care institutions require information to manage the quality of care provided and to allocate resources (e.g., labor, supplies, equipment, and facilities) according to the institution's patient case mix. Managers of provider institutions seek to link financial and patient care information to develop meaningful budgets, measure productivity and costs, and evaluate market position. Long-term institutional planning for personnel recruitment, equipment acquisition, and facilities development depends on anticipated trends in patient population needs.

Quality assurance activities constitute another information need. Such activities are a requirement for accreditation of hospitals by the Joint Commission on Accreditation of Healthcare Organizations (JCAHO); in addition, third-party payers carry out various quality monitoring and evaluation efforts. The best known is probably the Medicare peer review organization program administered by the Health Care Financing Administration (IOM, 1990c). Public and private third-party payers, medical professional societies, and researchers have been exploring practice guidelines and outcomes management as tools for improving care (IOM, 1990a,b). The risk management programs established by many health care institutions in response to the recent history of medical malpractice litigation add another level of information use (IOM, 1990c).

Patient care information to adjudicate claims for reimbursement made to third-party payers is an additional area of data needs. As expenditures related to health care have risen[10] and as third-party payers have sought to

---

[10]Health care expenditures accounted for 7.3 percent of the nation's gross national product (GNP) in 1970 (Levit et al., 1990). In 1989, health care spending amounted to 11.6 percent of GNP (U.S. Department of Health and Human Services, 1990).

contain costs, payers have also increased their demands for data. Patient data now are used for coverage decisions (e.g., preadmission review) as well as for payment. Cost-containment approaches such as utilization management rely on individual patient data for making short-term decisions; they also rely on aggregated data to make judgments about the effectiveness of medical services in the long term (IOM, 1989). A recently developed hybrid of quality assurance and cost containment—"value purchasing"—refers to the effort by purchasers, providers, and consumers to promote "the idea of value or quality within the context of cost" (IOM, 1990c:36). Value purchasing requires access to information on both costs and outcomes of care.

The public health arena is also seeking more and better data. The 1988 IOM report on the future of public health recommended that a uniform national data set be established to permit valid comparison of local, state, and national health data to facilitate progress toward achieving national health objectives (IOM, 1988). More recently, the U.S. Public Health Service identified public health surveillance as a primary means of supporting the national disease prevention objectives for the year 2000 (U.S. Public Health Service, 1990). Data are needed to understand the health status of the U.S. population and to develop, administer, and evaluate public health programs aimed at controlling and preventing adverse health events. The Public Health Service report specifically mentions data on (1) mortality, morbidity, and disability from acute and chronic conditions; (2) injuries; (3) personal, environmental, and occupational risk factors associated with illness and premature death; (4) preventive and treatment services; and (5) costs.

The issues of quality, cost, effectiveness, and appropriateness largely frame the questions that today's clinical and health services researchers pursue. Efficacy and safety are no longer sufficient criteria for assessing a technology whose purchasers also want to know (1) whether it is effective and safe outside the controlled environment of clinical trials, (2) whether it is cost-effective, and (3) whether it produces desired outcomes. "[L]ongitudinal observations of natural variations in use and outcomes of economically and clinically important medical technologies in different practice situations" are sought to support utilization management (IOM, 1989:158).[11]

Late in 1989, the Omnibus Budget Reconciliation Act (P.L. 101-239) established the Agency for Health Care Policy and Research (AHCPR) to enhance "the quality, appropriateness, and effectiveness of health care services, and access to such services, through the establishment of a broad

---

[11]One expert has suggested that "[w]hat is needed is a new kind of trial, one that combines randomized prescription of approved drugs and hands-off follow-up with recording of medical outcomes and determination of costs from routinely generated computerized patient records" (Paterson, 1988:112).

base of scientific research and through the promotion of improvements in clinical practice and in the organization, financing and delivery of health care services" (U.S. Congress, 1989). In addition to its mandate to "conduct and support research, demonstration projects, evaluations, training, and the dissemination of information, on health care services and on systems for the delivery of such systems," AHCPR is specifically directed to support the improvement and supplementation of existing databases and the design and development of new databases for use in outcomes and effectiveness research.

More recently, several IOM studies have endorsed efforts to support, expand, and improve research and the knowledge base on efficacy, effectiveness, and outcomes of care (IOM, 1990b,c). Such efforts are part of a systematic endeavor to develop clinical practice guidelines and standards of care. All of these activities underscore the vastly increased demand for patient data that has emerged during the 1980s.

Maintaining Confidentiality

In contrast to these trends—an increased supply of and demand for patient data—is the absolute necessity to protect patient privacy.[12] The ancient principle of confidentiality—the obligation of health care professionals to avoid violating a patient's right to privacy—is affirmed by the American Medical Association (AMA) Council on Ethical and Judicial Affairs (1989).[13] Thus, a significant challenge in creating future patient record systems is to achieve an appropriate balance between confidentiality and access by users with a need to know.[14]

---

[12]*Privacy* is the right of individuals to be left alone and to be protected against physical or psychological invasion or the misuse of their property. It includes "freedom from intrusion or observation into one's private affairs; the right to maintain control over certain personal information; and the freedom to act without outside interference" (Peck, 1984).

[13]"And whatsoever I shall see or hear in the course of my profession, as well as outside of my profession in my intercourse with men, if it be what should not be publicized abroad, I will never divulge, holding such things to be holy secrets" (Hippocratic Oath, as quoted in Small, 1989).

According to the AMA, "[t]he information disclosed to a physician during the course of the relationship between physician and patient is confidential to the greatest extent possible. The patient should feel free to make a full disclosure of information to the physician in order that the physician may most effectively provide needed services. The patient should be able to make this disclosure with the knowledge that the physician will respect the confidential nature of the communication" (AMA Council on Ethical and Judicial Affairs, 1989:21).

[14]Concerns about the privacy of information are not limited to health care data. The 1977 report, *Personal Privacy in an Information Society*, cited consumer credit, depository, insurance, employment, and education data as all needing protection (Privacy Protection Study Commission, 1977).

INFORMATION MANAGEMENT OPPORTUNITIES

Some health care provider institutions are well on their way toward developing new electronic approaches to patient records. This progress has been possible because of advances in computer technology and successful research on the application of such technology to medicine. These advances include, but are not limited to, hand-held computers; picture archiving and communications systems that permit electronic storage, transmission, and display of medical images; disk drives that offer mean time between failures of 60,000 or more hours; and high-speed telecommunications networks that can carry 1.7 billion characters per second over a 100-kilometer link. New technologies and applications such as these can potentially improve the quality of patient care, advance the scientific basis of medicine, moderate the costs of health care services, and enhance the education of health care professionals.

Computer-based patient records, as defined by the committee, could positively affect the quality of patient care in at least four ways. First, they offer a means of improving both the quality of and access to patient care data. Second, they allow providers to integrate information about patients over time and between settings of care. Third, they make medical knowledge more accessible for use by practitioners when needed. Fourth, they provide decision support to practitioners.

Research efforts could also benefit from computer-based patient record keeping in two key ways. First, improved data and access to those data would be available to researchers. Second, research findings could be communicated to practitioners through computer-based patient record systems.

Computer-based patient records could assist efforts to moderate the costs of health care in three ways. First, improved information could reduce redundant tests and services that are performed in response to the unavailability of test results. Second, administrative costs could be reduced by electronic submission of claims and the ability to generate routine reports automatically. Third, the productivity of practitioners could be enhanced by (1) reducing the time needed to find missing records or to wait for records already in use; (2) reducing, if not eliminating, the need for redundant data entry; and (3) reducing the time needed to enter or review data in records that have been streamlined to eliminate unnecessary information.

Health care professionals not only encourage self-directed learning among their students (Gastel and Rogers, 1989) but are viewed as having a responsibility for continuing lifelong education (AAMC, 1984). Students thus require skills in organizing information and solving problems. Computer-based patient records can support information management and independent learning by health care students and professionals in both patient care and clinical research settings. Tools for such learning include clinical decision support systems, bibliographic and knowledge links (including links to clinical practice guidelines), and statistical software.

BEYOND TECHNOLOGY

Meeting the challenge of managing health care information depends on more than technological advances. The usefulness of any technology depends on how well it and its progeny are applied. In addition to technology, a study of the improvement of patient records must address how the *use* of those records might be improved, a question that raises potentially sensitive issues.[15] "Improving records" and "improving clinical reasoning" are topics inevitably connected to one another because ideally the record reflects the clinical reasoning process. If better record systems are to be created in the future, the user must be recognized as part of the system, and the problem-solving activities of practitioners must be examined.

In addition to technological and behavioral opportunities for improving patient records, certain strategic issues must be addressed. Other information-intensive industries (e.g., banking) have successfully implemented widespread computer-based information management technologies. Understanding the factors that have slowed the development and diffusion of such technologies in health care is a first step toward achieving more rapid advances in the future.

WHY NOW?

Many attempts have been made over the years to advance clinical computing, to reform the patient record, and to encourage health care professionals to maintain the record more conscientiously (e.g., by entering necessary clinical data). Why should or how could renewed efforts to establish the routine use of new computer-based record systems succeed now when previous attempts have failed? Why might this report have a significant impact?

The committee believes that five conditions of the environment in which its strategic plan might be implemented increase the likelihood of achieving widespread use of computer-based patient records. First, current demands for patient information throughout the health care sector will not diminish; indeed, they will probably increase. Second, technologies essential to computer-based patient records are becoming more powerful and less expen-

---

[15]Examination of the role of patient records in the clinical process, as manifested in the debate surrounding the problem-oriented record, has been under way for more than 20 years (Weed, 1968; Goldfinger, 1972; Margolis, 1979).

sive. Third, patients and practitioners gradually are becoming accustomed to the use of computers in virtually all facets of everyday life. Fourth, an aging and mobile population results in more information to be managed and demands for improved transferability or portability of that information. Finally, the committee believes that those components of needed reform in health care that require evaluation, consolidation of data, and improved communication will not easily be achieved without reforms in the scope, use, and automation of the patient record.

REFERENCES

AAMC (Association of American Medical Colleges). 1984. *Physicians for the Twenty-first Century.* Report of the Panel on the General Professional Education of the Physician. Washington, D.C.: AAMC.

Amatayakul, M., and A. R. Sattler. 1990. Computerization of the medical record: How far are we? *Proceedings of the Fourteenth Annual Symposium on Computer Applications in Medical Care.* Los Alamitos, Calif.: IEEE Computer Society Press.

Amatayakul, M., and M. J. Wogan. 1989. Fundamental Considerations Related to the Institute of Medicine Patient Record Project. Paper prepared for the Institute of Medicine Committee on Improving Patient Records in Response to Increasing Functional Requirements and Technological Advances.

American Medical Association Council on Ethical and Judicial Affairs. 1989. *Current Opinions.* Chicago, Ill.: American Medical Association.

Barnett, O. 1990. Computers in medicine. *Journal of the American Medical Association* 263:2631-2633.

Bentsen, B. G. 1976. The accuracy of recording patient problems in family practice. *Journal of Medical Education* 51:311.

Bronson, D. L., A. S. Rubin, and H. M. Tufo. 1978. Patient education through record sharing. *Quality Review Bulletin* December:2-4.

Brook, R. H. 1989. Practice guidelines and practicing medicine: Are they compatible? *Journal of the American Medical Association* 262:3027-3030.

Burnum, J. F. 1989. The misinformation era: The fall of the medical record. *Annals of Internal Medicine* 110:482-484.

Case, C. L., and L. H. Jones. 1989. Continuity of care: Development and implementation of a shared patient data base. *Cancer Nursing* 12:332-338.

Covell, D. G., G. C. Uman, and P. R. Manning. 1985. Information needs in office practice: Are they being met? *Annals of Internal Medicine* 103:596-599.

Davies, A. R. 1990. Health Care Researchers' Uses and Requirements of the Patient Record. Unpublished draft memorandum to the Users and Uses Subcommittee of the Institute of Medicine Committee on Improving Patient Records in Response to Increasing Functional Requirements and Technological Advances. March.

Davies, A. R., and J. E. Ware. 1988. Involving consumers in quality assessment. *Health Affairs* 7:33-48.

Dawes, K. S. 1972. Survey of general practice records. *British Medical Journal* 3:219-223.

Donnelly, W. J. 1988. Righting the medical record: Transforming chronicle into story. *Journal of the American Medical Association* 260:823-825.

Ellwood, P. M. 1988. Shattuck Lecture—Outcomes management: A technology of patient experience. *New England Journal of Medicine* 23:1549-1556.

Feinstein, A. R. 1970. Quality of data in the medical record. *Computers and Biomedical Research* 3:426-435.

Fox, L. A., G. Stearns, and W. Imbiorski. 1979. *The Administrator's Guide to Evaluating Records and the Medical Record Department,* ed. The Beacon Group. Chicago, Ill.: Care Communications.

Fries, J. F. 1974. Alternatives in medical record formats. *Medical Care* 12:871-881.

GAO (General Accounting Office). 1991. *Medical ADP Systems: Automated Medical Records Hold Promise to Improve Patient Care.* Washington, D.C.: GAO.

Gardner, E., and L. Perry. 1989. Assessing computer links' risks and rewards. *Modern Healthcare* November 24:20-22, 26, 28.

Garrett, L. E., Jr., W. E. Hammond, and W. W. Stead. 1986. The effects of computerized medical records on provider efficiency and quality of care. *Methods of Information in Medicine* 25:151-157.

Gastel, B., and D. E. Rogers. 1989. *Clinical Education and the Doctor of Tomorrow.* Proceedings of the Josia Macy, Jr., Foundation National Seminar on Medical Education: Adapting Clinical Medical Education to the Needs of Today and Tomorrow. New York: New York Academy of Medicine.

Gerbert, B., and W. A. Hargreaves. 1986. Measuring physician behavior. *Medical Care* 24:838-847.

Goldfinger, S. E. 1972. The problem-oriented record: A critique from a believer. *New England Journal of Medicine* 288:606-608.

Greenes, R. A., and E. H. Shortliffe. 1990. Medical informatics: An emerging academic discipline and institutional priority. *Journal of the American Medical Association* 263:1114-1120.

Haynes, R. B., M. Ramsden, K. A. McKinnon, C. J. Walker, and N. C. Ryan. 1989. A review of medical education and medical informatics. *Academic Medicine* 64:207-212.

Hershey, C. O., M. H. McAloon, and D. A. Bertram. 1989. The new medical practice environment: Internists' view of the future. *Archives of Internal Medicine* 149:1745-1749.

Hsia, D. C., W. M. Krushat, A. B. Fagan, J. A. Tebbutt, and R. P. Kusserow. 1988. Accuracy of diagnostic coding for Medicare patients under the prospective-payment system. *New England Journal of Medicine* 318:352-355.

Huffman, E. K. 1981. *Medical Record Management.* Berwyn, Ill.: Physicians' Record Company.

IOM (Institute of Medicine). 1980. *Reliability of National Hospital Discharge Survey Data.* Report of a study. Washington, D.C.: National Academy of Sciences.

IOM. 1988. *The Future of Public Health.* Washington, D.C.: National Academy Press.

IOM. 1989. *Controlling Costs and Changing Patient Care? The Role of Utilization Management,* ed. B. H. Gray and M. J. Field. Washington, D.C.: National Academy Press.

IOM. 1990a. *Clinical Practice Guidelines: Directions for a New Program*, ed. M. J. Field and K. N. Lohr. Washington, D.C.: National Academy Press.

IOM. 1990b. *Effectiveness and Outcomes in Health Care*, ed. K. A. Heithoff and K. N. Lohr. Washington, D.C.: National Academy Press.

IOM. 1990c. *Medicare: A Strategy for Quality Assurance*, vols. 1 and 2, ed. K. N. Lohr. Washington, D.C.: National Academy Press.

Korpman, R. A., and T. L. Lincoln. 1988. The computer-stored medical record: For whom? *Journal of the American Medical Association* 259:3454-3456.

Kurland, L. T., and C. A. Molgaard. 1981. The patient record in epidemiology. *Scientific American* 245:54-63.

Levit, K. R., M. S. Freeland, and D. R. Waldo. 1990. National health care spending trends: 1988. *Health Affairs* 9:171-184.

Lindberg, D. A. B. 1979. *The Growth of Medical Information Systems in the United States.* Lexington, Mass.: Lexington Books.

MacEachern, M. T. 1937. *Medical Records in the Hospital.* Chicago, Ill.: Physicians' Record Company.

Mamlin, J. J., and D. H. Baker. 1973. Combined time-motion and work sampling study in a general medicine clinic. *Medical Care* 11:449-456.

Margolis, C. Z. 1979. Problem-oriented record: A critical review. *Paediatrician* 8:152-162.

Martin, J. B. 1990. The environment and future of health information systems. *Journal of Health Administration Education* 8:11-24.

National Institutes of Health. 1989. *National Library of Medicine MEDLARS: The World of Medicine at Your Fingertips.* NIH Pub. No. 89-1286. Bethesda, Md.: U.S. Department of Health and Human Services.

Paterson, M. L. 1988. The challenge to technology assessment: An industry viewpoint. Pp. 106-125 in *Quality of Care and Technology Assessment*, ed. K. N. Lohr and R. A. Rettig. Washington, D.C.: National Academy Press.

Peck, R. S. 1984. Extending the constitutional right to privacy in the new technological age. *Hofstra Law Review* 12:893-912.

Pories, W. J. 1990. Is the medical record dangerous to our health? *North Carolina Medical Journal* 51:47-55.

Privacy Protection Study Commission. 1977. *Personal Privacy in an Information Society.* Washington, D.C.: U.S. Government Printing Office.

Richart, R. H. 1970. Evaluation of a medical data system. *Computers and Biomedical Research* 3:415-425.

Rogers, J. L., and O. M. Haring. 1979. The impact of a computerized medical record summary system on incidence and length of hospitalization. *Medical Care* 6:618-630.

Rogers, J. L., O. M. Haring, P. M. Wortman, R. A. Watson, and J. P. Goetz. 1982. Medical information systems: Assessing impact in the areas of hypertension, obesity and renal disease. *Medical Care* 20:63-74.

Romm, F. J., and S. M. Putnam. 1981. The validity of the medical record. *Medical Care* 19:310-315.

Rulin, M. C., T. T. Hayashi, and D. M. Badway. 1988. Continuity of ambulatory care in an obstetrics and gynecology residency program. *Obstetrics and Gynecology* 71:787-790.

Saba, V. K., D. M. Oatway, and K. A. Rieder. 1989. How to use nursing information sources. *Nursing Outlook* 37:189-195.

Small, S. A. 1989. Confidentiality issues for health administrators. *Hospital and Health Services Administration* 34:591-598.

Shortliffe, E. H., L. E. Perreault, L. M. Fagan, and G. Wiederhold, eds. 1990. *Medical Informatics Computer Applications in Health Care*. Reading, Mass.: Addison-Wesley Publishing Company.

Tarlov, A. R., J. E. Ware, A. Greenfield, E. C. Nelson, E. Perrin, and M. Zubkoff. 1989. The Medical Outcomes Study: An application of methods for monitoring the results of medical care. *Journal of the American Medical Association* 262:925-930.

Tufo, H. M., and J. J. Speidel. 1971. Problems with medical records. *Medical Care* 9:509-517.

Tufo, H. M., R. E. Bouchard, A. S. Rubin, J. C. Twitchell, H. C. VanBuren, and L. Bedard. 1977. Problem-oriented approach to practice. 2. Development of the system through audit and implication. *Journal of the American Medical Association* 237:502-505.

U.S. Congress. 1989. *Congressional Record*, vol. 135, no. 165 (pt. 3). November 21.

U.S. Department of Health and Human Services. 1990. *HHS News*. December 20.

U.S. Public Health Service. 1990. *Healthy People 2000: National Health Promotion and Disease Prevention Objectives*. DHHS Pub. No. (PHS) 90-50212. Washington, D.C.: U.S. Department of Health and Human Services.

Weed, L. L. 1968. Medical records that guide and teach. *New England Journal of Medicine* 12:593-600, 652-657.

Westin, A. F. 1976. *Computers, Health Records and Citizen Rights*. National Bureau of Standards Monograph No. 157. Washington, D.C.: U.S. Government Printing Office.

Whiting-O'Keefe, Q. E., D. W. Simborg, W. V. Epstein, and A. Warger. 1985. A computerized summary medical record system can provide more information than the standard medical record. *Journal of the American Medical Association* 254:1185-1192.

Zimmerman, J. 1978. *Physician Utilization of Medical Records: Preliminary Determinations*. St. Louis, Mo.: Washington University, Biomedical Computer Lab.

Zuckerman, A. E., B. Starfield, C. Hochreiter, and B. Kovasznay. 1975. Validating the content of pediatric outpatient medical records by means of tape-recording doctor-patient encounters. *Pediatrics* 56:407-411.

2

The Computer-Based Patient Record: Meeting Health Care Needs

In recent years, computerization of patient records has increased at a moderate rate and this trend is likely to continue, particularly as technology improves and becomes more affordable and as the demand for health care information increases. If future patient records are merely automated versions of most current records, however, an opportunity to improve a fundamental resource for health care will have been lost. For example, in the patient record of the future, the committee seeks the ability to access quickly a list of current problems, a trail of clinical logic, the patient's health status, and the most recent information about various treatment options for the patient's condition. Easy access to and sound organization of data elements can be provided by automation of patient records, but the availability of the data elements depends on whether practitioners collect and record such data in the first place. Further, access to bibliographic and knowledge databases will require new functions not provided by traditional patient records.

Thus, the automation of patient record retrieval, maintenance, and use is necessary, but not sufficient, for record improvement. Given existing and emerging computer technologies and the evolving nature of health care, the committee believes that the patient record can, must, and will develop to meet the expanding needs of the health care field. This chapter identifies the attributes of future patient records that are required to meet these needs, discussing several of them in detail to highlight the scope and complexity of the issues to be addressed.

DEFINING HEALTH CARE NEEDS

The quality of a patient record or a patient record system depends on its ability to meet the needs and requirements of those who use it. As discussed below, those users include, but are not limited to, physicians and nurses delivering care to patients. The committee followed three steps suggested by the continuous quality improvement model to develop its vision of an improved patient record and record system: (1) identify the customers; (2) understand their requirements; and (3) translate those requirements into functional characteristics of the system (Donabedian, 1966, 1988; Batalden and Buchanan, 1989; Berwick, 1989).[1]

Patient Record Users

The committee broadly defined the users of patient records as those individuals who enter, verify, correct, analyze, or obtain information from the record, either directly or through an intermediary. All users of the patient record ultimately support patient care. They differ, however, in how and why they use the record.

Some users have daily contact with the record, others access the record sporadically, and still others never actually handle the record but rely on data derived from it. An exhaustive list of patient record users would essentially parallel a list of the individuals and organizations associated directly or indirectly with the provision of health care. Patient record users provide, manage, review, or reimburse patient care services; conduct clinical or health services research; educate health care professionals or patients; develop or regulate health care technologies; accredit health care professionals or provider institutions; and make health care policy decisions. All of these kinds of users are "customers" of the patient record, and their needs should be met by patient record systems of the future.

Users are individuals, but they most commonly perform their functions on behalf of institutions. Boxes 2-1A and 2-1B identify types of individuals and organizations that rely on patient records or the data they contain. These lists are illustrative rather than comprehensive and indicate the wide range of users and settings in which patient records are employed.

The full array of patient record users and the respective needs of each were too extensive for the committee to address fully. Therefore, it identified five major categories of users that it considered the most significant and representative. Specifically, the committee focused on practitioners (phy-

---

[1]As stated by Juran (1989), the remaining steps of the quality improvement process are as follows: (4) design a system capable of supplying these functional characteristics; (5) implement the design; (6) prove the value of the system; and (7) stabilize or further improve the system, depending on the results of ongoing evaluation. Given the scope of its charge, the committee stopped short of designing such a system; it did, however, accomplish an intermediate step by determining the technological implications of the functional requirements of future patient record systems (see Chapter 3).

BOX 2-1A   REPRESENTATIVE INDIVIDUAL USERS OF PATIENT RECORDS

Patient Care Delivery (Providers)

Chaplains
Dental hygienists
Dentists
Dietitians
Laboratory technologists
Nurses
Occupational therapists
Optometrists
Pharmacists
Physical therapists
Physicians
Physician assistants
Podiatrists
Psychologists
Radiology technologists
Respiratory therapists
Social workers

Patient Care Delivery (Consumers)

Patients
Families

Patient Care Management and Support

Administrators
Financial managers and accountants
Quality assurance managers
Records professionals
Risk managers
Unit clerks
Utilization review managers

Patient Care Reimbursement

Benefit managers
Insurers (federal, state, and private)

Other

Accreditors
Government policymakers and legislators
Lawyers
Health care researchers and clinical investigators
Health sciences journalists and editors

---

sicians, nurses, and other health professionals), patients, administrators, third-party payers, and researchers.[2]

Patient Record Uses

Just as the range of patient record users includes more than physicians, nurses, and other health care professionals, patient record uses extend beyond direct patient care. Similar to a comprehensive list of users, a complete list of uses would be quite long. Boxes 2-2A and 2-2B list examples of primary and secondary uses of patient records.

---

[2]Setting priorities among patient record users risks giving the needs of some users too little consideration or possibly omitting them entirely. Uncomfortable with this compromise, the committee remained acutely aware that designers and implementers of future patient record systems must attend to the needs of all parties, not just those discussed in detail in this report.

Primary uses of patient records are associated with the provision of patient care, that is, with providing, consuming, managing, reviewing, supporting, and charging and reimbursing patient care services. Secondary uses of patient records are not considered necessary for a particular encounter between a patient and a health care professional, but such uses influence

---

BOX 2-1B   REPRESENTATIVE INSTITUTIONAL USERS OF PATIENT RECORDS

Health Care Delivery (inpatient and outpatient)
Alliances, associations, networks, and systems of providers
Ambulatory surgery centers
Donor banks (blood, tissue, organs)
Health maintenance organizations
Home care agencies
Hospices
Hospitals (general and specialty)*
Nursing homes
Preferred provider organizations
Physician offices (large and small group practices, individual practitioners)
Psychiatric facilities
Public health departments
Substance abuse programs

Management and Review of Care
Medicare peer review organizations
Quality assurance companies
Risk management companies
Utilization review and utilization management companies

Reimbursement of Care
Business health care coalitions

Employers
Insurers (federal, state, and private)

Research
Disease registries
Health data organizations
Health care technology developers and manufacturers (equipment and device firms, pharmaceutical firms, and computer hardware and software vendors for patient record systems)
Research centers

Education
Allied health professional schools and programs
Schools of medicine
Schools of nursing
Schools of public health

Accreditation
Accreditation organizations
Institutional licensure agencies
Professional licensure agencies

Policymaking
Federal government agencies
Local government agencies
State government agencies

*Various hospital departments are one kind of institutional patient record user. A few such users include the blood bank, diagnostic radiology, emergency medical services, intensive care units, nutrition services, pharmacy, surgery, and social work.

BOX 2-2A   PRIMARY USES OF PATIENT RECORDS

Patient Care Delivery (Patient)
Document services received
Constitute proof of identity
Self-manage care
Verify billing

Patient Care Delivery (Provider)
Foster continuity of care
   (i.e., serve as a communication tool)
Describe diseases and causes
   (i.e, support diagnostic work)
Support decision making about
   diagnosis and treatment of
   patients
Assess and manage risk for
   individual patients
Facilitate care in accordance
   with clinical practice guidelines
Document patient risk factors
Assess and document patient
   expectations and patient
   satisfaction
Generate care plans
Determine preventive advice or
   health maintenance
   information
Remind clinicians (e.g., screens,
   age-related reminders)
Support nursing care

Document services provided
   (e.g., drugs, therapies)

Patient Care Management
Document case mix in institu-
   tions and practices
Analyze severity of illness
Formulate practice guidelines
Manage risk
Characterize the use of services
Provide the basis for utilization
   review
Perform quality assurance

Patient Care Support
Allocate resources
Analyze trends and develop
   forecasts
Assess workload
Communicate between departments

Billing and Reimbursement
Document services for payments
Bill for services
Submit insurance claims
Adjudicate insurance claims
Determine disabilities (e.g.,
   workmen's compensation)
Manage costs
Report costs
Perform actuarial analysis

the environment in which patient care is provided. Education, research and development, regulation, and policymaking are all considered secondary uses of the patient record.

Practical considerations forced the committee to focus on certain high-priority record uses rather than on all possible functions of the record. The four major categories of patient record uses considered by the committee were direct patient care, administration and management, reimbursement, and research.

TRANSLATING CUSTOMER NEEDS INTO SYSTEM REQUIREMENTS

Proper system design means achieving a patient record system that properly fits, interacts with, and communicates in the accepted manner of every user community the system supports. This kind of design is necessary if automated patient record systems are to be adopted by users. The committee defined the needs of patient record users in terms of system function and issues of implementation and operation. System function is what the system enables users to do and what it does for them. Implementation and operation issues relate to the factors users consider in acquiring and installing a system. These factors are important regardless of the form of the record (e.g., paper or computer-based).

The specific features users seek in patient records and record systems are described below in terms of the computer-based patient record (CPR). Most of these desired features are common to two or more major kinds of record users. Unique concerns or needs of a user group are also identified. Box 2-3 presents an overview of user requirements.

BOX 2-2B SECONDARY USES OF PATIENT RECORDS

Education
Document health care professional experience
Prepare conferences and presentations
Teach health care professions students

Regulation
Serve as evidence in litigation
Foster postmarketing surveillance
Assess compliance with standards of care
Accredit professionals and hospitals
Compare health care organizations

Research
Develop new products
Conduct clinical research

Assess technology
Study patient outcomes
Study effectiveness and cost-effectiveness of patient care
Identify populations at risk
Develop registries and databases
Assess the cost-effectiveness of record systems

Policy
Allocate resources
Conduct strategic planning
Monitor public health

Industry
Conduct research and development
Plan marketing strategy

BOX 2-3 USER REQUIREMENTS FOR PATIENT RECORDS AND RECORD SYSTEMS

Record Content
Uniform core data elements
Standardized coding systems
and formats
Common data dictionary
Information on outcomes of
care and functional status

Record Format
"Front-page" problem list
Ability to "flip through the record"
Integrated among disciplines and
sites of care

System Performance
Rapid retrieval
24-hour access
Available at convenient places
Easy data input

Linkages
Linkages with other information
systems (e.g., radiology,
laboratory)
Transferability of information
among specialties and sites
Linkages with relevant scientific
literature
Linkages with other institutional
databases and registries
Linkages with records of family
members

Electronic transfer of billing
information

Intelligence
Decision support
Clinician reminders
"Alarm" systems capable of being
customized

Reporting Capabilities
"Derived documents" (e.g.,
insurance forms)
Easily customized output and
other user interfaces
Standard clinical reports (e.g.,
discharge summary)
Customized and ad hoc reports (e.g.,
specific evaluation queries)
Trend reports and graphics

Control and Access
Easy access for patients and their
advocates
Safeguards against violation of
confidentiality

Training and Implementation
Minimal training required for
system use
Graduated implementation
possible

In compiling the list of user requirements, the committee noted two special considerations. First, user needs can conflict with each other—not just *among* groups (e.g., patients and practitioners need confidentiality, but claims payers seek access to detailed clinical information), but also *within* a single user group (e.g., doctors want access to information to be very fast, but they may also want to be able to sort information according to complicated logical rules, which slows response times). To the extent possible, the committee resolved such conflicts by using sensible rules of priority. In several cases, however, the conflicts remained nettlesome and are discussed in Chapter 4 as particular challenges to future patient record development.

Second, at a technological frontier, customers may have difficulty expressing or even imagining a need. This situation may well occur with the computer-based patient record, which contains opportunities for functional characteristics that most users would not think to request. The pioneering designer must not only ask, "What do people want?" but also, "What would people want if they knew what could be done for them?"

Patient Record Functions

The traditional function of patient records has been to store information relevant to the care of a patient for subsequent retrieval. Patient record systems should offer users at least two additional functions. First, records should be able to guide the process of clinical problem solving. Second, records should support clinicians with decision analysis, reminders, risk assessment, and other "intelligent" features not available with paper records.

Storage

The attributes associated with the storage function are record access (i.e., availability, convenience, speed, and ease of use), quality, security, flexibility, connectivity, and efficiency.

ACCESS   First and foremost, users want to retrieve information easily when and where they need it. Other features of a patient record system are essentially irrelevant to users if they cannot gain access to the system, to the records in the system, or to the data in the records.

Access can be described in terms of availability, convenience, reliability,[3] and ease of use. A patient record system should allow authorized clinical users convenient access to any record 24 hours a day. This requirement implies an adequate number of conveniently located terminals or workstations, no system downtime, no lost records or data, and access to the record by more than one user at the same time. Nonclinical users typically require access to patient record data at least during standard working hours.

Different users need different levels and kinds of information (see Box 2-4). The ease with which users locate or retrieve needed data elements depends largely on the record format. Current paper record formats tend to segregate rather than integrate information; to facilitate communication of

---

[3]*System reliability* refers to the constant availability of hardware and software needed for work in the clinical setting.

needed information, an integrated format is necessary. Thus, records should contain a front-page problem list to allow users to locate desired information. In addition, record systems should allow users to "flip through" or easily scan records; a table of contents or index would be helpful for this purpose.

BOX 2-4 DIFFERENT USERS NEED DIFFERENT LEVELS AND KINDS OF DATA

A patient record database contains many data elements, and each user community has a unique, definable "view" of the database that brings together the elements needed by that community. (Some communities also have specialized or occasional views for special circumstances.) Some views overlap, and some data elements appear in many views. Other data elements appear only in one view.

For each view that supports a given user community, processes are needed to organize its contents, manipulate and display it in various ways, and allow users to commingle views. System-level processes that automatically support all views (e.g., calendar-date management, screening for access authorization to maintain confidentiality) are also required.

For example, in a teaching hospital:

- The general internist wants a view that will help him or her manage the medical aspects of the case.
- The subspecialist's view must contain additional details relevant to his or her special duties in a case.
- The chief resident needs additional details to support teaching during rounds.
- The intensive care nurse needs a view that embraces the care and management of the patient to whom he or she is assigned.
- The pharmacy's view supports patient medication, including medication history and patient response to drugs.
- The dietitian requires a view to support diet and nutrition control for the patient.
- The security department's view identifies security risks or hazardous patients.
- The accounting department has a view relating to what should be charged.
- A research view permits academic researchers to access data without violating confidentiality.
- Multiple reporting views are required to prepare internal or external reports for policymakers as appropriate.

Several other capabilities are needed for optimal access. Users should be able to display information at different levels of detail. Moreover, the system should permit virtually every data item to be used as a key for retrieval and should also enable users to access subsets of data. All users, regardless of their level of computer expertise, should be able to enter most queries without the intervention of a programmer; thus, an English-like retrieval language should be part of the system.

Accessing information when needed includes more than finding an available terminal; from the user's point of view, it means an adequate (i.e., fast) system response time. Users want to perform their tasks at least as fast as they currently perform them with paper records. Extremely rapid retrieval of information, measured in fractions of a second, is an essential function for primary users of the CPR. In addition, clinicians, who are accustomed to writing or dictating their entries to patient records, want a comparable method in the CPR system to add data to the record.

From the users' perspective, the difficulty involved in learning to use a system also affects access. Thus, operation of patient record systems should require only minimal training.[4] Training for physicians in particular should be short and easy, preferably occurring "on line" and at their convenience. Many physicians are unwilling to devote large blocks of time to learning a new record system, even if ultimately it might make their work easier. In addition, built-in, displayable "help" documentation on system operation and the data elements should be available to both clinical and nonclinical users.

The question of patient access to records is debated among practitioners. It is likely, however, that the trend toward increasing patient access will continue. Some providers consider it appropriate for patients to enter data (e.g., historical medical information) into their records routinely. Recently, functional status and preferences among various treatments have been identified as data that could be recorded by patients to assist practitioners in developing care plans.

Some practitioners encourage patients to audit their records for accuracy and completeness; they may also use the record for patient education. Indeed, as patients become increasingly computer-literate, knowledge-seeking consumers of health care services, the CPR may function as an important patient education tool by offering patients access to resources such as MEDLINE.

---

[4]This statement assumes that record users will receive adequate training in how to use patient records and the other functions provided by patient record systems through formal education (i.e., professional schools and continuing education). It also refers to the requirement that users who work in more than one provider setting (e.g., physician office and hospital) be able to learn multiple patient record systems easily.

DATA QUALITY The notion of data quality has several attributes: legibility, accuracy, completeness, and meaning. CPR systems eliminate the need for handwriting and thus improve legibility. Accuracy of CPRs can be enhanced by data-entry screens and logical rules that flag or block inappropriate entries for particular data fields. To the extent that CPRs reduce the need for an intermediary to enter data (i.e., for transcription), a potential source of errors (and cost) is removed. When errors do occur, for legal purposes the original entry and the correction should both be preserved (Waller, in this volume). Data accuracy also has implications for the security and reliability of CPR systems insofar as the systems must ensure that data are not lost or unknowingly corrupted.[5]

The completeness of patient records for subsequent users depends in part on agreement among users about uniform core data elements. Without such uniformity, what one patient record user views as complete data may be considered incomplete by another. Data completeness implies that systems will accommodate the currently expected range and complexity of clinical data and that they will permit new data fields to be added and obsolete data fields to be identified.[6]

For patient records to meet user needs, patient problems and the current status of patient problems should be clearly noted in the record. In addition, it is essential that the health care provider's rationale for clinical decisions be clearly documented. Lack of a recorded rationale hinders the ability of subsequent users of the record to make appropriate judgments regarding patient care, quality assurance, utilization review, reimbursement, and research.

For purposes of health services research, patient health status is the single most important data element that is usually missing from the patient records of today. Formal, interpretable information on health status is a precondition both to case-mix or risk-factor adjustment and to assessment of the outcomes of care. The research community clearly wants health status information, collected in a standard format, to be a routine part of the record of the future. Such records should also document health risk factors (e.g., smoking).

Technology assessment, clinical investigation, and health services research have been slowed by the lack of reliable, valid, standardized, consis-

---

[5]The term *corrupted* is used to describe data that do not accurately represent the information they are intended to reflect (e.g., data that have been transposed, scrambled, or omitted).

[6]After a period of time, certain data elements in a record or record system may no longer be used to collect new information. Currently obsolete data elements are nevertheless legitimate data elements in the old records, and they should be retained as long as old records are retrieved and used.

tently collected information on the health status and functional level of patients (Ellwood, 1988; Roper et al., 1988). Moreover, practitioners may benefit from routine availability of health status measures. Some evidence suggests that without such measurements in routine clinical practice, physicians and other health care professionals often overlook significant impairments and changes in function among their patients (Nelson, 1990). In the past two decades, many health services researchers have worked to develop, test, and refine health status measures with sound psychometric characteristics (Katz, 1987; Lohr and Ware, 1987; McDowell and Newell, 1987; Lohr, 1989). These kinds of methodological advances could greatly increase the practical application of standardized health status data.

The committee acknowledged that the question of whether and how soon health status assessment will influence the quality of care remains to be addressed. To gain a better understanding of the value of health status measures, the committee supported their widespread adoption as a component of the patient record—but under conditions that would permit evaluation of whom they help and of how best they can be employed. The committee did not identify an optimal set of health status measurement instruments, as this determination was not part of its charge. Rather, to broaden the base of potential comparisons of case mix, care, morbidity, and outcomes, the committee noted the potential value of standardizing or otherwise increasing the compatibility of those instruments now in common use.

It remains unclear how outcome data can be gathered and used unobtrusively, inexpensively, and conveniently enough that such activities will become widespread. Merely adopting a computerized record format may not overcome the barriers that so far have impeded the diffusion of health status measurement into routine clinical practice. Computerization may make the analysis of such information easier but may not affect its collection.

The completeness of patient records depends in part on the time it takes to add new information to the record, once that information is available. Data completeness can be enhanced by linkages between CPR systems and ancillary systems (e.g., laboratory, radiology), which permit the transfer of results from ancillary systems to the CPR in the hospital, physician's office, or other provider setting as soon as such results are available.

Maintaining the quality of patient data also requires that the data have meaning for users. Effective retrieval and use of information from patient records depend on consistency in naming or describing the same findings, clinical problems, procedures, drugs, and other data within a single patient record, across many patient records in a single record system, or in other systems that contain data relevant to the understanding and treatment of patient problems. Communication among practitioners can be aided by a common clinical data dictionary and a clinical coding system that are interchangeable any clinical data common to different specialists or professions but specific enough to describe the detailed data unique to a profession or specialty.

Health care researchers have a special need for record systems that provide more uniform results than are provided by current systems. Consistent description of clinical content becomes more important with the aggregation of data from many patient records—as in outcomes research, for example. Standardized data dictionaries, coding schemes, and uniform data sets permit more complete, reliable analyses of care and disease patterns involving multiple sites.[7]

SECURITY   CPR systems have two security requirements. First, as discussed in Chapter 1, patient and provider privacy must be protected. Second, data and software must be safeguarded against tampering and unintentional destruction. These requirements demand both system and data security measures. *System security* refers to the measures taken to keep computer-based information systems safe from unauthorized access and other harm. *Data security* involves protection of data from accidental or intentional disclosure to unauthorized persons and from unauthorized alteration.

Data security includes both data confidentiality and data integrity. *Data confidentiality* is a "requirement whose purpose is to keep sensitive information from being disclosed to unauthorized recipients" (National Research Council [NRC], 1991:52). Confidentiality requires appropriate action by physicians, nurses, midwives, secretaries, medical technicians, paramedical staff, social workers, hospital managers, computer staff, and research investigators in health care facilities to safeguard the privacy of patient information. Confidentiality also requires that computer systems refuse access to unauthorized individuals.

In its narrowest sense, *data integrity* refers to the consistency and accuracy of data stored in computer-based systems. It is a "requirement meant to ensure that information and programs are changed only in a specified and authorized manner" (NRC, 1991:54). Data integrity is of paramount importance to the CPR, and care must be taken, especially in distributed CPR systems (see Chapter 3), to ensure that records can be completely restored in the event of system failures.

A broader definition of data integrity could also be appropriately applied to patient data. Data are said to have integrity if they comply with an a priori stated expectation that they have a defined set of attributes. This a

----

[7]The difficulties associated with establishing standardized data dictionaries and coding schemes should not be underestimated. Synonyms with unique mapping specifications across terms and codes may provide an interim solution until full-fledged standard dictionaries and codes can be developed.

priori set of attributes is unique to the data, to the process operating on the data, and to the data holder. Such attributes might include timeliness (e.g., every data element is posted within five minutes of availability), complete-ness (e.g., a certain set of data elements must be part of the record), and accuracy (e.g., there are no spelling errors, every address has a zip code).

Data integrity in future patient records might be enhanced by including a *data validity* field that would flag data that might not be correct. Data validity would be an additional parameter against which integrity could be judged and thereby controlled. Informing subsequent users that an entry might be incor-rect would allow them to discount or ignore the information.

FLEXIBILITY Users assign high priority to flexibility in records; they do not want to be forced to use the record in a universally uniform or pre-scribed manner. Thus, future CPR systems should permit customization of data-entry formats, reporting formats, and display formats—both for and, in some cases, by specific users. Patient record user needs are simply too many and too varied for any one combination of input, reporting, or display options. Furthermore, research has shown that the ability to customize computer interfaces according to one's preferences and work habits increases user acceptance of computer systems (Bikson et al., 1987).

Conventional formats should be designed and available as default modes, but the users of the patient record of the future should find the record easy to mold to their individual, local needs. Different formats for displaying infor-mation on the screen or on paper should be available. The record should also permit integration across disciplines and professional specialties and pro-vide different "views"[8] of patient data for different users (see Box 2-4).

Flexibility is also required to meet the varied reporting needs of users, particularly physician specialties. Doctors need record information avail-able both in easily accessible, standard reporting formats (such as letters, insurance forms, school and camp certificates, etc.) and in formats they can easily customize according to specialty and individual taste. Therefore, the CPR system should contain a user-friendly report generator for physicians and others who wish to design specialized reports for their own use.

CONNECTIVITY Connectivity denotes the potential of the record or record system to establish links or to interact effectively with any sort of provider

---

[8]The term *view* has a special use in computer science. A view is considered to be perspective on a database. Different users of a database may have different uses for and therefore different perspectives on the same database. For example, some users may require data elements that are not of interest to other users. Alternatively, different users may seek the same data elements presented in different formats (e.g., as a table or a graph showing trends) or may want several data elements combined to create a new data element.

or database that may improve the care of the patient. Three different interfaces are important in such interactions: the interface among records or record systems of different provider institutions, the interface between the record and other repositories or potential repositories of information that may be useful in caring for the patient, and the interface between the record and a practitioner.

Linkages among the various clinical records pertaining to a single patient are also important to users, who often want a *longitudinal* patient record—records from different times, providers, and sites of care that are linked to form a lifelong view of a patient's health care experiences. Linkages are also needed to transfer patient data from one care setting to another (e.g., from physician office to hospital) to facilitate service coordination.

Linking the records of family members, or the records of individuals who received a certain procedure in a particular facility, may prove useful for some types of epidemiological analysis. The aggregation of patient data for large-scale analysis, however, requires more complicated kinds of linkages. Integration of relevant subsets of data across institutional boundaries is especially important as researchers attempt to understand diseases and episodes of illness independent of the particular institution or health care professional with whom patients find themselves at a particular phase of their illness.

Patient record systems should also offer linkages to other databases and other sources of information.[9] Desirable linkages include databases that contain scientific literature and bibliographic information, administrative information (e.g., coverage for a particular elective procedure for a given insurance plan), medical practice guidelines, insurance claims, and disease registries.

Connectivity makes several other demands on the system as well. To make it simple for the practitioner to interact with the record, data entry must be almost as easy as writing, and databases must be organized in such a way that any terminal or microcomputer on the system can retrieve requested data. As noted earlier, communication among practitioners depends on common data dictionaries and clinical coding systems. To interface easily with a database or registry requires a different sort of connectivity. Workstations must be designed with telecommunications interfaces that allow the user to switch almost instantly between the information in the record and its relevant counterpart in the external knowledge base.

---

[9]Outbound linkages (i.e., linkages in which information is transmitted to a remote location) create additional concerns about maintaining confidentiality and require adequate network security as well as adequate system security.

EFFICIENCY Users want to minimize expense, effort, complexity, and waste. To achieve such efficiencies, computer-based patient record systems must include certain capabilities—in particular, one-time data entry and performance of routine tasks. Further, CPR systems should be designed so that data content is streamlined and unnecessary data are not collected.

Any data entered into the system should be available for a variety of uses, eliminating the need for redundant data entry. (The need for manual extraction of data and re-entry procedures greatly diminishes the value of a system.) The system should be designed to ensure that data are available to support patient care, organizational operations, and decision making. Thus, data must be viewed as an organizational resource, not property "owned" or controlled by the departments that happen to collect them or that are the primary users of the data.

The CPR system should be a part of an integrated patient care information system. If the system is hospital based, it should communicate with systems in the clinical laboratory, pharmacy, respiratory therapy, other ancillary services, referring physician offices, and other care settings (e.g., home, nursing home) so that data will not require manual transcription from one system to another. If the system is based in a physician's office, it should communicate with the computer systems of local clinical laboratories, pharmacies, hospitals, and other physicians' offices.[10]

CPR systems should facilitate the movement of data into, within, and outside of the automated patient record. In particular, they should permit raw and aggregated data to be moved to another electronic database for further analysis and storage. For example, a hospital or individual physician should be able to extract selected information electronically from a patient care database to send to other internal or external (perhaps national) databases.[11] In addition, the system should have no trouble accepting data directly from electronic monitoring devices and other patient care equipment.

Health care professionals perform many routine administrative tasks in the course of providing services, and they seek ways to reduce this administrative burden so that they can devote more time to direct patient care, research, and education. Patient record systems should provide the capacity to generate routine documents based on record data automatically, to submit insurance claims electronically, and to report adverse reactions or occurrences of tracked diseases automatically.

Computer-based records must be designed to avoid the mere replication

---

[10]Requiring such communication within and between institutions increases the complexity of achieving adequate security measures to maintain confidentiality.

[11]This data transmittal capability assumes that adequate security measures are in place.

of paper record features and behaviors that, upon reflection, have little or no value to users. Examples of waste include information that is routinely collected but never used; inflexible, redundant formats for recording data that result in duplicative information (e.g., obsolescent manual medication files); and retrospective quality assurance that could be replaced with on-line quality assurance. Such features and behaviors add cost rather than quality to the record system.

The committee did not specifically investigate the nature or scope of such wasted effort in present-day records, but members shared the general impression that it abounds. In developing the CPR, time would be well spent in practical research to identify and remove these "non-value-added" steps, features, and data elements, with the intent of producing a record that is leaner, less complex, and more streamlined than that of today. This process is likely to require changes in regulations or laws, and the committee urges that such changes be analyzed, recommended, and adopted (see Chapter 5).

Guidance of Clinical Problem Solving

It has been suggested that a physician's thought process is formed in part by his or her interaction with the patient record (Young, 1987). According to Weed (1968), a properly formatted patient record can guide clinicians through the process of clinical problem solving. It was this intention that led Weed to design the problem-oriented medical record (POMR) (Weed, 1968; Margolis, 1979).[12]

Studies investigating the use of the problem-oriented format to record the patient care process report three advantages over non-problem-oriented

---

[12]The problem-oriented medical record categorizes clinical information relevant to the medical care of the patient into four functional groups. *Clinical data* include demographic data, subjective data provided by the patient as clinical history, and objective data elicited either by physical examination or by technical means (e.g., laboratory tests, radiology examinations). *Clinical problem data* are grouped by levels of specification, which may be defined (in increasing order of sophistication) as symptoms, signs, abnormal laboratory data, pathophysiologic states, and diagnoses. Problem definition is essential to organizing much of the data in the record. Problems should be defined at a level of specification appropriate for the data available and should be described in both objective and subjective terms. Psychosocial problems should also be identified. *Planning data* are different from the above two kinds of data in that they are determined by the provider and patient after the baseline clinical data have been collected and the clinical problems have been defined. Three basic sorts of data for planning patient management are diagnostic, therapeutic, and patient education plans. Plans should be linked clearly to the relevant clinical problem. Finally, *follow-up data* are generated any time after initial plans have been implemented. The main types of follow-up data are new subjective data, objective data, the provider's assessment of these data, and new plans.

(i.e., source-oriented or other) formats. First, the chance of follow-up for a problem listed in the problem list is significantly greater (Simborg et al., 1976; Starfield et al., 1979). In other words, the POMR's front-page problem list is a particularly useful feature. Second, it is easier to relate information in the record to a relevant problem (Aranda, 1974). Third, the format reflects an orderly process of problem solving, a heuristic that aids in identifying, managing, and resolving patients' problems (Weed, 1968).

The committee unanimously believes that patient records should guide and reflect clinical problem solving and that the mere translation of current record formats, data, and habits from paper to computer-based systems will not alone produce the range of improvements in care potentially achievable in a truly reformed patient record system. Current systems include behaviors and record forms that produce substantial waste, imprecision, and complexity in a care system less and less able to tolerate that burden. The committee also believes that the shift from a paper to a computer-based system offers an opportunity to study and improve clinical approaches and methods that are reflected in the record. Some formats are likely to be more effective than others in guiding and encouraging the use of an efficient, scientific problem-solving method in the clinical process.

The committee did not reach unanimity regarding the choice of a single preferred record format to support improved clinical care. A majority maintained that no clearly superior alternative existed to warrant specific recommendation; this group therefore concluded that, at present, the primary pertinent requirement of a CPR is that it be sufficiently flexible to accommodate a wide range of present and future record formats.

Although it did not specifically recommend use of the POMR, the committee did consider certain components of the POMR to be highly desirable in any computer-based record system. Those components include (1) a structured, systematically collected database; (2) an easily reviewed and updated problem list; and (3) routine recording of clinical formulations and plans for care and follow-up. The committee urges continuing research to develop, design, and assess improved record formats that, over time, are likely to be used more consistently throughout the health care system.

A minority of committee members maintained that one patient record format—the problem-oriented medical record first described by Weed—offers a superior alternative in guiding and supporting scientific reasoning and clear communication in medical practice. Those who favored the POMR format argued that it is a general model that rests on a firm theoretical foundation and that its slow diffusion over the past two decades reflects in part practical barriers that may be overcome in a computer-based record environment. They recommended that clinicians use the POMR unless a specific alternative format is preferred in a particular practice setting.

Practitioner Support

Given the volume and complexity of the information required to provide patient care, users want the patient record to be more than a repository of data. Computer-based record systems can support practitioners by providing at least five kinds of tools that are not available with paper records. These tools include mechanisms for focusing attention, for patient-specific consultation, for information management, for data analysis, and for implementing quality assurance and cost management policies.

Human cognition has measurable limitations, and as a result humans "predictably overlook rare and uncommon events" (McDonald and Tierney, 1988:3435). Automated record systems can help practitioners recognize out-of-range values or dangerous trends, remember needed actions, recall available options, and make better clinical decisions. Human memory is imperfect, especially when the task involves remembering a large set of items or recalling the same items repeatedly. The computer can be relied on to remember large numbers of items accurately and to check routinely whether the practitioner has forgotten any standard items relevant to the diagnosis or treatment of a particular problem. Some of these reminders may be critical, and they can be linked to alarms (such as beep tones or messages) that warn the practitioner before trouble occurs.[13] (For example, an alarm might be triggered when two incompatible drugs are prescribed together.)

CPR systems can also provide easy access to clinical decision support systems that provide "custom-tailored assessments or advice based on sets of patient-specific data" (Shortliffe et al., 1990: 469). Currently available patient-specific consultation systems suggest differential diagnoses, indicate additional information that would help to narrow the range of etiologic possibilities, suggest a single best explanation for a patient's symptoms, or provide advice on therapy (Shortliffe et al., 1990).

CPR systems can support practitioners in the patient care setting by providing easy access to knowledge and bibliographic databases. Such access will free practitioners from relying on memory for infrequently used information. Moreover, computer-based record systems can help educate practitioners and keep them up-to-date on new developments by providing access

---

[13] As discussed in Chapter 4, a significant factor to be addressed in CPR system development and implementation is the need for system users to change certain behaviors. The availability of reminders in either preventive or emergency situations will require practitioners to change their behavior; as a result, such reminders may not at first be embraced warmly by practitioners. Indeed, the value of this technology must be sufficiently demonstrated before practitioners will change their behavior.

to bibliographic information when they need it (Association of American Medical Colleges, 1986; Haynes et al., 1989).

CPR systems can provide descriptive, graphical, and statistical analyses of clinical data using standard statistical software packages. In addition, CPR data can be rearranged and analyzed for ongoing quality assessment and to provide physicians and patients with quantitative assessments of the risks of conditions and treatments. (These assessments would promote formal decision analysis of many problems that at present cannot benefit from such analysis because of the lack of required data.) CPR system capabilities can facilitate these tasks in several ways: (1) rapid searching through single or multiple records; (2) sorting information in one record or information aggregated across multiple records; (3) aggregating data across patients by hospital, patient care unit, and department; and (4) allowing easy abstraction of information throughout patients' hospital stays or episodes of care.

Finally, CPR systems should offer practitioners and health care managers a means for implementing quality assurance and cost-management policies at the time and site of care (Barnett et al., 1978; Barton and Schoenbaum, 1990; Tierney et al., 1990). CPR systems can also be a resource for guiding policies and practice by providing analysis of past clinical experience within a provider setting (McDonald and Tierney, 1988).

Implementation and Operation Issues

Managers of health care organizations are faced with ever-increasing demands for data. From outside their organizations, requests come from regulators, payers, and community interest groups, among others; from inside their institutions, inquiries come from researchers and those responsible for utilization management and quality assurance. These managers are well aware that few existing record systems can meet these demands. They also recognize, and are wary of, both the cost and the conflict that may be incurred if they attempt to introduce major changes in record systems. Many institutions lack the capital for a sudden conversion to new computer architectures. Even if the funds were available, however, some managers are concerned that physician-management relationships, already strained in many medical organizations, could be further disrupted by an institution's insistence that physicians accept a new method or pattern of record keeping.

Nevertheless, administrators generally seem to prefer that the patient record not be frozen in its present form. They seek to implement change to a new system in a phased sequence, so that it can be more easily managed. Most user groups, but especially institutional managers, will have trouble implementing a vastly modified record system all at once. Proper design of advanced systems must involve well-considered plans for phasing in the changes that are going to be made. Otherwise, provider institutions in particular will feel extended beyond their financial and organizational capabilities.

THE FUTURE PATIENT RECORD

The promise of significantly improved health care through the technological capabilities of computers constitutes the basis for the committee's vision of future patient records and patient record systems. The committee offers this vision to help readers picture what such records and systems can do and to serve as a standard against which current and future CPR systems can be compared.

Future patient records will have many more users and uses than present records. Direct providers of care (physicians, nurses, dentists, and other health care professionals) will remain the users of highest priority in design considerations. The needs of all users, however, can be accommodated to an extent not possible in current record systems.

The committee identified five objectives for future patient record systems. First, future patient records must support patient care and improve its quality. Second, they must enhance the productivity of health care professionals and reduce the administrative and labor costs associated with health care delivery and financing. Third, they must support clinical and health services research. Fourth, they must be able to accommodate future developments in health care technology, policy, management, and finance. Fifth— and the committee placed great emphasis on this—patient confidentiality must be maintained while these objectives are being met.

In the patient record of the future, the entire notion of such a record will be broadened from that of a location or device for keeping track of patient care events to that of a resource with much enhanced utility in patient care, management of the health care system, and extension of knowledge. Properly designed and used, the record will provide an accurate longitudinal account of care. The record system will also be broadened to include functions beyond those available in current record systems; it will help to improve care by reminding, linking, and guiding health care professionals and organizations. In short, the record of the future will be an asset in managing and improving the care of patients.

In the past, the basic function of a patient record was to store patient data for use by those involved in patient care. Even this classic function will be broader in the future, however, especially with respect to the key feature of flexibility. Different health care professionals require record information to be retrieved and displayed in different formats. Today, both paper and computer records are often cumbersome tools for information retrieval and display. The record of the future will be far more flexible and will permit users to design and utilize reporting formats tailored to their special needs.

Future patient records will provide new dimensions of record functionality through links to other databases, decision support tools, and reliable transmission of detailed information across substantial distances. To meet the needs of practitioners, future patient record systems will be linked to knowledge bases, clinical decision support systems, statistical software packages, and video or picture graphics. In hospitals, various departmental systems (e.g., finance, laboratory, nursing, radiology) will be able to communicate with the patient record system. Physician offices will be able to communicate with local hospitals and with national bibliographic resources such as MEDLINE. In the larger health care environment, computer-based information management systems will be able to communicate with information systems of provider institutions, third-party payers, and other health care entities.

As noted in the committee's definition of a patient record system, *people* are also a system component. Optimal functioning of future systems poses four conditions for users. First, they must have confidence in the data (which implies that data must be entered directly by the practitioner who collected it, reliably integrated among all sources, and accurately retrieved whenever needed). Second, they must use the record actively in the clinical process. Third, they must understand that the record is a resource for studying the effectiveness and efficiency of clinical processes, procedures, and technologies. Fourth, they must be capable of using future computer-based record systems efficiently.

The committee visualizes the CPR as the core of health care information systems. Figure 2-1 illustrates the various types of interactions in which CPR systems will be required to engage. Such systems must be able to transmit data to other types of clinical and administrative information systems within provider institutions; they must also be able to transmit data to other provider institutions or to secondary databases. (For example, CPR systems in physicians' offices should be able to communicate with local hospitals.) In addition, CPR systems must also be able to accept data from other internal and external computer-based systems.

Figure 2-2 illustrates the committee's vision of a national health care information system. Such a system would support the transmission of data for clinical purposes and, with appropriate confidentiality measures, for reimbursement and research purposes. It would also bring information resources (e.g., MEDLINE) to virtually all practitioners. A national health care information system would require that local, regional, and national networks be established. These networks would provide the means to transmit a laboratory report from a hospital to a physician's office or to send a patient record across the country. A national health care information system with these and other capabilities could support the coordination and integration of health care services across settings and among providers of care.

Intrainstitutional Sources or	External Sources or
Recipients of Patient Data	Recipients of Patient Data
Patient (or family)	Other provider institutions
Individual practitioners	hospitals
Clinical services and departments	nursing homes
laboratory	physicians' offices
nursing	Other patient care settings
pharmacy	inpatient
radiology	outpatient (including home health)
Administrative, management, and support services	Secondary patient records
and departments	educational institutions for the health
admitting	professions
finance	quality assurance and accreditation agencies
risk management	registries and databases
	researchers
	state and local public health agencies
	third-party payers

FIGURE 2.1   Computer-based patient records as the core of health care information systems.

   In delineating its vision of a national health care information system, the committee is not proposing that a single CPR system be imposed on health care providers; indeed, no single CPR system is likely to meet the wide range of CPR user needs.   Imposing a single system on health care providers is likely to result in the loss of desirable flexibility.   Moreover, there is no mechanism for accomplishing such a task in the pluralistic health care system of the United States.   Nevertheless, the committee believes all CPR systems must meet minimum connectivity requirements and offer a set of standard functions.   To accommodate various user communities and institutions, however, the committee anticipates that a range of CPR systems will be available.   For example, CPR systems will offer a range of additional functions and come in a variety of sizes; they will also have varying price tags, depending on individual provider requirements.   In other words, the committee seeks a national transportation system for patient data.   The transportation system will require an infrastructure (e.g., networks) and standards for connectivity and security but will retain a substantial amount of flexibility.

   The notion of a health care information system should not suggest that all patient data will be collected in a monolithic database.   Rather, CPR data

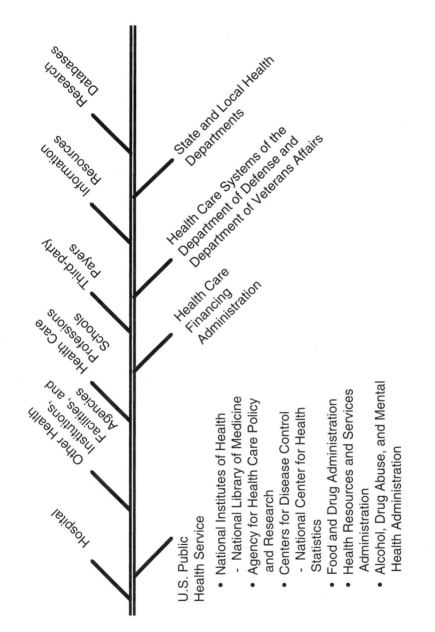

FIGURE 2.2 Computer-based patient records as part of a national care information system.

should be collected so that they can produce quality secondary records; subject to appropriate controls, these records can be added to institutional, local, regional, national, or international databases as needed for clinical, administrative, or research purposes.

In summary, the committee believes that the computer-based patient record can play an increasingly important role in the health care environment. This role begins in the care process by providing patient information when needed and by supporting clinical decision making. It extends to the management of care by establishing a mechanism by which quality assurance procedures and clinical practice guidelines (including the most recent warnings on contraindications and adverse reactions to therapies) can be brought to health care professionals at the time and site of patient care. It also includes providing opportunities for reducing administrative costs associated with health care financing and collecting administrative data for internal and external review. It encompasses enhancing health care professional education by supporting independent, lifelong learning. Finally, it extends to capturing relevant, accurate data necessary for technology assessment, health services research, and related studies concerning the appropriateness, effectiveness, and outcomes of care.

REFERENCES

Aranda, J. M.   1974.   The problem-oriented medical records: Experiences in a community hospital. *Journal of the American Medical Association* 229:549-551.

Association of American Medical Colleges. 1986. *Medical Education in the Information Age: Proceedings of the Symposium on Medical Informatics.* Washington, D.C.

Barnett, O. G., R. Winickoff, J. L. Dorsey, M. M. Morgan, and R. S. Lurie. 1978. Quality assurance through automated monitoring and concurrent feedback using a computer-based medical information system. *Medical Care* 16:962-970.

Barton, M. B., and S. C. Schoenbaum. 1990. Improving influenza vaccination performance in an HMO setting: The use of computer-generated reminders and peer comparison feedback. *American Journal of Public Health* 80:534-536.

Batalden, P. B., and E. D. Buchanan. 1989. Industrial models of quality improvement. Pp. 133-159 in *Providing Quality Care: The Challenge to Clinicians*, ed. N. Goldfield and D. B. Nash, D.B. Philadelphia, Pa.: American College of Physicians.

Berwick, D. M. 1989. Sounding board: Continuous improvement as an ideal in health care. *New England Journal of Medicine* 320:53-56.

Bikson, T. K., B. A. Gutek, and D. A. Mankin. 1987. *Implementing Computerized Procedures in Office Settings: Influence and Outcomes.* Santa Monica, Calif.: The RAND Corporation.

Donabedian, A. 1966. Evaluating the quality of medical care. *Milbank Memorial Fund Quarterly* 44(pt. 2):166-203.

Donabedian, A. 1988. The quality of care. How can it be assessed? *Journal of the American Medical Assocation* 260:1743-1748.

Ellwood, P. M. 1988. Shattuck lecture—Outcomes management: A technology of patient experience. *New England Journal of Medicine* 23:1549-1556.

Haynes, R. B., M. Ramsden, K. A. McKibbon, C. J. Walker, and N. C. Ryan. 1989. A review of medical education and medical informatics. *Academic Medicine* 64: 207-212.

Juran, J. M. 1989. *Juran on Quality Planning.* New York: McGraw-Hill.

Katz, S., ed. 1987. The Portugal conference: Measuring quality of life and functional status in clinical and epidemiological research. *Journal of Chronic Diseases* 40:459-650.

Lohr, K. N., ed. 1989. Advances in health status assessment: Conference proceedings. *Medical Care* 27(suppl.):S1-S294.

Lohr, K. N., and J. E. Ware, Jr., eds. 1987. Proceedings of the Advances in Health Assessment Conference. *Journal of Chronic Diseases* 40(suppl. 1):1S-193S.

Margolis, C. Z. 1979. Problem-oriented record: A critical review. *Paediatrician* 8:152-162.

McDonald, C. J., and W. M. Tierney. 1988. Computer-stored medical records: Their future role in medical practice. *Journal of the American Medical Association* 259:3433-3440.

McDowell, I., and C. Newell. 1987. *Measuring Health: A Guide to Rating Scales and Questionnaires.* New York: Oxford University Press.

Nelson, E. C. 1990. Using outcomes measures to improve care delivered by physicians and hospitals. Pp. 201-211 in *Effectiveness and Outcomes in Health Care,* ed. K. A. Heithoff and K. N. Lohr. Washington, D.C.: National Academy Press.

NRC (National Research Council). 1991. *Computers at Risk: Safe Computing in the Information Age.* Washington, D.C.: National Academy Press.

Roper, W. L., W. Winkenwerder, G. M. Hackbarth, and H. Krakauer. 1988. Effectiveness in health care: An initiative to evaluate and improve medical practice. *New England Journal of Medicine* 18:1197-1202.

Shortliffe, E. H., L. E. Perreault, L. M. Fagan, and G. Wiederhold, eds. 1990. *Medical Informatics Computer Applications in Health Care.* Reading, Mass.: Addison-Wesley Publishing Company.

Simborg, P. W., B. H. Starfield, and S. D. Horn. 1976. Information factors affecting problem follow-up in ambulatory care. *Medical Care* 14:848-856.

Starfield, B., D. Steinwachs, I. Morris, G. Bause, S. Siebert, and C. Westin. 1979. Concordance between medical records and observations regarding information on coordination of care. *Medical Care* 17:758-766.

Tierney, W. M., M. E. Miller, and C. J. McDonald. 1990. The effect on test ordering of informing physicians of the charges for outpatient diagnostic tests. *New England Journal of Medicine* 322:1499-1504.

Weed, L. L. 1968. Medical records that guide and teach. *New England Journal of Medicine* 12:593-600, 652-657.

Young, D. W. 1987. What makes doctors use computers? Discussion paper. Pp. 8-14 in *Use and Impact of Computers in Clinical Medicine,* ed. J. G. Anderson and S. J. Jay. New York: Springer-Verlag.

3

Computer-Based Patient
Record Technologies

User needs, both of individuals and of cohesive communities, are paramount in the design and development of computer-based patient record systems. Designers and vendors of CPR systems must understand such needs, as well as how the systems will be used and what demands users will place on the systems. The discussion of user requirements in Chapter 2 sets the stage for explaining in this chapter the attributes of technologies required to create CPR systems in the 1990s.

This chapter has three main goals: (1) to highlight technologies relevant to CPR systems, (2) to convey what is possible with existing technologies, and (3) to emphasize what will be required to build state-of-the-art CPR systems in the 1990s. The chapter also provides some insight into the current state of existing clinical information systems that possess features crucial to the development of state-of-the-art CPR systems. Finally, it discusses the technological barriers that still must be overcome before CPR systems can become well established.

TECHNOLOGICAL BUILDING BLOCKS FOR CPR SYSTEMS

No clinical information system in 1990 is sufficiently comprehensive to serve as a complete model for future CPR systems. That is, no operational clinical information system in 1990 can manage the entire patient care record with all its inherent complexities. A few existing clinical information systems are beginning to approach the CPR system capabilities envisioned by the committee. None of these is yet complete, but some might appropriately be called today's CPR systems. Therefore, the committee sometimes refers to current CPR systems, meaning those clinical information systems that are beginning to approximate the ideal CPR system envisioned by the committee for the future (see Chapter 2).

The committee selected and reviewed nine technologies that are significant for CPR systems. They include (1) databases and database management systems, (2) workstations, (3) data acquisition and retrieval, (4) text processing, (5) image processing and storage, (6) data-exchange and vocabulary standards, (7) system communications and network infrastructure, (8) system reliability and security, and (9) linkages to secondary databases. This section describes the key attributes of these crucial technologies.

Databases and Database Management Systems

It is important to distinguish between the clinical data—that is, the computer-based patient record, or CPR—and the system that captures and processes those data—that is, the CPR system. *CPR* functions relate to the collection of data, such as patients' medical problems, diagnoses, treatments, and other important patient information, including follow-up data and quality measures. *CPR system* functions relate to storage capacity, response time, reliability, security, and other similar attributes, but the system relies on the collection of clinical data, the core CPR, to support virtually all of its activities.

Databases

The most desirable database model for CPR systems involves either (1) a distributed database design—that is, a system with physically distributed computers and databases but with logical central control of the entire record; or (2) a centrally integrated physical database design—that is, a centrally located, complete CPR within a single computer-stored database (see Figure 3-1);[1] or (3) some hybrid or mix of these two approaches. In any case, the key requirements are central control and organizational integrity of the entire record for each individual patient. Central control permits authorized persons using a terminal located anywhere in the information system to access the entire integrated patient record or any of its parts, regardless of the locations of any other departmental subsystems where the various data items may have originated. (Access is allowed only on the basis of parameters specific to authorized users.)

---

[1]The selection of the database management system that undergirds a CPR system is critical to the performance and success of the system. Several publications during the past decade have discussed this issue: Barnett et al. (1982); Pryor et al. (1983), Wiederhold (1986), Kirby et al. (1987), McDonald et al. (1988), Whiting-O'Keefe et al. (1988), Wilton and McCoy (1989), Canfield et al. (1990), Friedman et al. (1990), and Hammond et al. (1990).

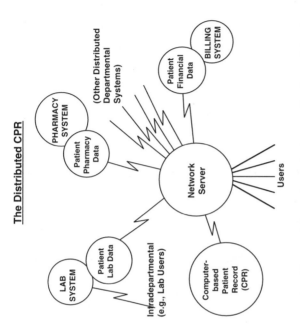

The Centralized CPR

In this model, all patient data are stored in the central CPR, which is the core of the CPR system. The CPR system may be complete, supporting laboratory and nearly all other departmental functions, or it may receive data from remote distributed departmental subsystems for purposes of maintaining a complete central CPR.

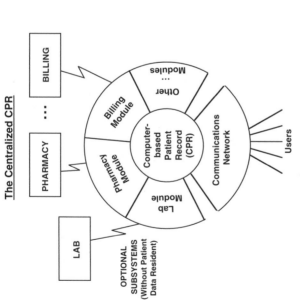

The Distributed CPR

In this model, patient data are distributed in departmental systems or subsystems. Consequently, the complete CPR does not exist in any one place; rather, portions of the record are distributed among several computer systems. A node on the network might regularly gather data from the distributed computers to present a "view" of the patient's complete CPR.

FIGURE 3-1 Centralized *vs.* distributed computer-based patient record.

Although the feasibility of the distributed database design (see the right-hand panel of Figure 3-1) has recently gained support from the development of networking technologies, most current clinical information systems that might qualify as CPR systems use a centralized design (the left-hand panel of Figure 3-1). The CPR systems of today cannot as yet acquire and retrieve all patient care data directly. Instead, they rely on data transmitted to the CPR system through interfaces with departmental subsystems; the data are subsequently entered into the CPR using applications programmed on the CPR system. One major factor that differentiates current CPR systems is the extent to which they use local area networks, or LANs, to access departmental subsystems and stand-alone databases containing portions of the CPR.

Today's CPR systems place great emphasis on providing at least a "view" of a complete, centralized patient record (Hammond et al., 1990). If the patient's clinical data are physically distributed among several computers in a network, a comprehensive view of the record of a given patient can be achieved only by retrieving and assembling the pertinent data from each computer on the network where patient data reside. Although this scenario has a number of advocates and some advantages, it also has several severe problems (Margulies et al., 1989; Hammond et al., 1990).

A careful analysis of the two contrasting models shown in Figure 3-1 may be helpful in understanding the main problems. In the distributed system, the patient record is physically distributed among several computer systems but at the same time is functionally integrated. This means that a variety of distributed patient care applications will generate and use patient care data in the distributed CPR. It also means that individual records may require multiple data structures (or data files), which tends to lengthen data retrieval times. Another problem with a distributed system is that data synchrony—that is, the correct sequencing of a patient's time-stamped data that are entered into the system at the same time but from different sources—must be guaranteed at both the applications and the database management system (DBMS) levels. Perhaps the most significant problem with the distributed database approach, however, is the increased potential it carries for circumventing CPR confidentiality mechanisms. Because portions of the patient's record are distributed among several different computers, ensuring confidentiality becomes more difficult. Every computer has its own vulnerabilities, and each one that is added to a network represents another node that must be protected and another potential entry point for unauthorized access (National Research Council, 1991).

Database Management Systems

A major technological issue is the complexity of the data that will eventually reside in the CPR. The CPR of the future will consist of many different kinds of data, including text, graphics, images, numerical data, sound, and full-motion video. To design a functionally integrated database system that accommodates such diversity is a sizable technical challenge.

The CPR is so complex that no single database management system is capable of optimally storing and retrieving the full range of patient data (Hammond et al., 1990). As a result, CPR system developers have used a variety of complementary DBMSs to address these complexities. This multiple-DBMS approach is most common when the CPR system uses the distributed database scenario; in that case, each subsystem often uses a different DBMS. Because the CPR is distributed across many connected subsystems, each subsystem will probably use a DBMS that is particularly suited to the kind of data most frequently stored in that subsystem. The collection of appropriate databases that results offers advantages of efficiency in manipulating and storing the CPR complex data. Some CPR system developers have even created their own proprietary database management systems, tailored to the CPR's particular complexities.

The selection or creation of the DBMS that will support the CPR is among the first and most crucial steps in developing a CPR system. Several database management systems or architectures have evolved in recent years. Four important ones developed by commercial vendors are hierarchical, relational, text-oriented, and object-oriented databases. Each of these architectures has its own particular strengths and weaknesses. Architects of current CPR systems (both commercial and private) have mainly used hierarchical, relational, or text-oriented models. Viable object-oriented database management systems have been introduced only recently and are not yet in widespread use.

Workstations

Three general classes of workstations seem likely to prevail in future CPR systems. First, "smart" terminals with data-entry pointer/selector devices (e.g., mouse, touch-screen, light-pen, or voice) will be used for data input and retrieval; they may also support "windowing" and medium-resolution imaging. These terminals will use a graphical user interface (GUI) and communicate with file servers, compute servers, and rule servers[2] in a local area net-

---

[2]As computers have become smaller, more powerful, and more affordable, individual computer systems have been dedicated to functions common to many applications and users in a network. For example, data files may be stored in a computer dedicated to serving the filing needs of network users, hence the name *file server*. Similarly, network users executing computationally intensive applications (e.g., three-dimensional reconstruction of images of an artery) require access to computers capable of serving rapid computation needs, hence the name *compute server*. Another commonly needed capability on a network is access to systems capable of rapidly executing rules for decision support, hence the name *rule server*. As medical decision support systems become more robust, rule servers will play an increasingly important role in health care networks.

work. Second, hand-held terminals or computers, or other similar semiportable devices, will facilitate either manual or voice entry of data into the CPR. These relatively portable devices will be used at the bedside by practitioners. Third, fully configured workstations (e.g., complete with a mouse, accelerated processors, GUI, and large storage capacities) may well become one of the more powerful tools ever devised for health care professionals and may ultimately come to be considered indispensable.

Data Acquisition and Data Retrieval

Data Acquisition

Data acquisition for the CPR remains an exceptionally challenging topic within the field of medical informatics.[3] Ideally, data in the CPR should be entered at its source (e.g., the site of patient care) by the record's primary user; they should be entered only once, and they should be accessible to all portions of the CPR system that use that particular data item. Data entry at the source by members of the health care team remains a sensitive issue. Yet the most commonly used alternative, data entry by an intermediary (e.g., a clerk or a transcriptionist) has several disadvantages: (1) it often introduces errors because the person who has direct information about the patient is not the person entering the data; (2) it delays the timely availability and transmittal of potentially critical information; (3) it makes immediate feedback to health care professionals (in the form of alerts or alarms generated by detectable errors or conflicting orders) impossible; and (4) it interferes with the decision maker's ability to use linked databases and other on-line knowledge bases designed to assist health care professionals in the clinical decision-making process. Two keys to the success of next-generation CPR systems are ease of use and proper incentives for data entry at the data source (Young, 1987; Safran et al., 1989).

Data Retrieval

The organization of data displays that can quickly convey crucial information needed in a particular setting (e.g., in the intensive care unit) or by a certain user (e.g., a surgeon) is also a challenge (Stead and Hammond, 1987; Silva et al., 1990). Because much of the patient record can be presented as text, tables, or graphs (e.g., trends in laboratory values), most CPR systems today display data on low-cost monitors capable of high-

---

[3]Greenes and Shortliffe (1990) define *medical informatics* as "the field that concerns itself with the cognitive, information processing, and communication tasks of medical practice, education, and research, including the information science and technology to support these tasks."

resolution graphics. Although these displays cannot deliver, for example, high-definition radiological images, they can produce hard-copy printouts of display screens, graphs and tables, and signals such as those needed for an electrocardiogram (ECG). A complete on-line CPR reduces the necessity for printing multipart copies of these printouts.

A short response time has proven to be an important factor in successful CPR systems (Bleich and Slack, 1989). This requirement refers primarily to retrieving data, but it is equally important for inputting data. In future CPR systems, the displays and reporting formats of CPR data are likely to be configured or modified by users. Thus, the same data may be presented differently, or in different combinations, to different health care professionals, each of whom has differing "views" or "windows" into the same CPR (see Chapter 2). Customizing data in this way is a difficult capability to implement but will produce a system that is much more attractive to end users.

Text Processing

To establish a diagnosis, physicians and other health care professionals use patient information in a textual form—for example, the patient history and the results of the physical examination. With a CPR system, professionals search for and retrieve such text from database systems using query languages, which in the past were often idiosyncratic to a particular system. In recent years, gradual progress has been made in standardizing such languages.

Natural-language understanding, or the ability of the computer system to selectively extract meaning from textual data, has been slower to evolve because of its inherently greater complexity (Obermeier, 1989). Compounding this complexity is the slow development of efforts to encourage a more uniform vocabulary in health care. Automated speech-recognition systems may help to add uniformity and consistency to vocabularies for the CPR by encouraging the speaker to use clinically relevant, yet consistent, terminology.

In the 1990s, text-processing systems for translating the narrative found in discharge summaries and other parts of the CPR are likely to be used to generate codes for billing. As text-processing systems improve in accuracy and performance, they may be used to extract significant phrases or attributes from the CPR that could assist the user in searching related databases. For example, attributes derived from the CPR might be matched against the terms and concepts in the National Library of Medicine's (NLM) Unified Medical Language System (UMLS; Humphreys and Lindberg, 1989). Improved text-processing systems would make it possible to use data from the CPR, in conjunction with the UMLS, to lead practitioners to an array of related information sources, including medical literature and other pertinent knowledge bases (Lindberg and Humphreys, 1990).

Image Processing and Storage

Medical imaging today includes diagnostic images or pictures obtained by film scanners, computed radiography (CR), magnetic resonance (MR), computed tomography (CT), ultrasound, and nuclear medicine sources. The medical images generated by these technologies and found in today's patient records are typically two-dimensional, still pictures. The increasing digitization of data, however, will expand the capabilities of such technologies. For example, digital data permit varying intensity resolution (number of measurable levels of gray), which allows the computer to display images with medium to high contrast. In the near future, digital images will be routinely available in many radiology departments.

New technological developments are expected to lead to a new generation of picture archiving and communications systems (PACSs), which will be installed in many radiology departments by the mid-1990s. PACSs permit the electronic storage, transmission, and display of medical images throughout a medical facility and offer many advantages not available with conventional film. For example, two or more physicians can simultaneously examine exact duplicates of an image at their respective and sometimes distant locations, discuss the interpretation of the image, and together formulate plans for optimal patient management. Imaging systems in the near future will eliminate concerns about the current status or location of an image, such as "missing" or "in transit."

Imaging is routinely used not only by radiologists but also by ophthalmologists, dermatologists, pathologists, dentists, and other specialists. Indeed, images have become an essential part of the complete patient record. Yet although the record is incomplete without images, the typical paper record environment stores images separately from the chart itself. CPR systems of the future, when appropriately linked to PACSs, will allow health care professionals to view images at the computer workstation in a timely fashion.

Data-Exchange and Vocabulary Standards

In today's health care environment, health care professionals, managers, policymakers, regulators, and educators need increasing amounts of accurate health care data in machine-readable form to support intelligent decision making. All such data must be collected, aggregated (when they come from diverse sources), and transmitted among disparate systems. The aggregation and dissemination of existing and future health care data mandate the development of standards, both to exchange health care data and to encourage more consistent medical vocabulary, especially in those portions of the CPR containing natural-language text. Developing such standards requires a coordinated approach.

Efforts to develop data-exchange standards for components of the CPR have only recently gained significant momentum in the United States. Because so much is at stake in this sizable medical market—a market that remains largely untapped from the vendors' point of view—standards take on an even more prominent role in fostering the evolution of the required technologies. Currently, there are several related efforts to standardize and facilitate the exchange of health data. HL 7 and Medix, as well as standards from the American Society for Testing and Materials (ASTM), the American College of Radiologists/National Electrical Manufacturers Association (ACR/NEMA), and others are representative of the current movement to formulate data-exchange standards.[4]

Several promising vocabulary developments are relevant to CPR systems. These include a planned new edition of the Systematized Nomenclature of Medicine (SNOMED); the Read Clinical Classification in Great Britain; the ASTM *Standard Guide for Nosologic Standards and Guides for Construction of New Biomedical Nomenclature*, which is now completed and ready for distribution (ASTM, 1989); and the NLM's UMLS project. The overall goal of UMLS is to help users retrieve relevant biomedical

---

[4]HL 7 is a specification for a health data-interchange standard designed to facilitate the transfer of health data resident on different and disparate computer systems in a health care setting. For example, HL 7 facilitates the transfer of laboratory results, pharmacy data, and other information for a patient to a central hospital system without concern for whether such systems are supplied by the same vendor or manufacturer. HL 7 is not, however, designed to support the transfer of the entire patient record. For example, it does not address the transfer of image data (such as those from a PACS).

The Institute of Electronic and Electrical Engineers (IEEE) has begun to develop Medix, a comprehensive health data-exchange standard. It is the only standard for which its developers have stated an objective of eventually supporting transfer of the entire patient record, although it is not yet mature enough to do so routinely in a health care setting. Medix is also the only health care data standard that has declared an intention to support the International Standards Organization's (ISO) Open Systems Interconnect (OSI) model.

ASTM has sponsored committees (e.g., E 31.12 and E 31.14) on computerized systems that are dedicated to standards directly related to the transfer of clinical data, such as those found in the patient record. Among other topics, these ASTM standards committees have focused on naming conventions and have proposed data element names for clinical data found in the patient record. They have also addressed specifications for transferring clinical laboratory data messages between independent computer systems.

ACR/NEMA have joined together to establish a functioning standard designed to transfer images between disparate computer systems (especially different PACSs).

information from multiple machine-readable sources, even though different vocabularies and classifications may have been used in these sources. One of the new knowledge sources being developed to support this goal is a metathesaurus, which will link related terms and concepts from a variety of existing biomedical vocabularies and classifications.

System Communications and Network Infrastructure

Caring for patients naturally requires many health care workers to interact frequently. As discussed in Chapter 2, health care is information intensive, which implies a strong emphasis on the communication and transmission of information to many people in diverse places. The patient information conveyed is complex and appears in all possible modalities, including text, images, voices and sounds, signals, and video. This broad array of information needs to be available in such diverse locations as the bedside, the hospital department, professional offices, emergency settings including mobile units, and the home.

Technologies to support communications of all kinds are evolving at an unprecedented rate. With the advent of fiber optics, in particular, transmitting the diversity of information contained in the CPR will soon be feasible at high speeds and low costs.

Of great significance is the evolving Integrated Services Digital Network (ISDN), an all-digital network capable of high-speed transmission of all modalities (data, voice, graphics, or video) over public telephone networks. In the 1990s, the transition from analog to fully digital switches is expected to occur throughout much of the United States. This transition to an all-digital network, when complete, will have wide-ranging implications for improving health care because it will open a new era for communication of all types of information, including that contained in the CPR.

System Reliability and Security

Chapter 2 presented brief explanations of system reliability, system security, and data security. System security is achieved through appropriate system design and the use of physical security measures directed toward protection of the computing environment and equipment. For example, techniques for security include software and hardware features, physical measures such as locks and badges, identification numbers or codes, passwords, and an informed, security-conscious staff (National Research Council, 1991).

A data integrity control policy has at least four essential components: (1) security measures, (2) procedural controls, (3) assigned responsibility, and (4) audit trails. It is especially important to allow access to the CPR system only to those with a need to know and to certify their identity before permitting access. In addition, the CPR system must be capable of providing different levels of data confidentiality as required for its various users. Audits of all legitimate users of CPR systems must be conducted regularly to remind and assure patients and staff that strict confidentiality is being maintained and measured. Such periodic audits should help deter any attempts by staff to breach confidentiality.

Members of the health care team who record patient data in the record are responsible for such entries, but in a hospital or clinic, physicians typically still have primary responsibility for ensuring the record's accuracy. As documentation of health care shifts from paper to computer-based records, practitioners will maintain their responsibility to document patient care, but the data will reside within CPR systems. Legal, professional, and accrediting standards must be revised to specify appropriate new roles and responsibilities associated with the shift from the paper chart to the CPR.

In the aggregate, current CPR systems seem to use limited measures for ensuring patient confidentiality. Most CPR systems do not approach the levels of security or confidentiality that airlines or banks, for example, maintain to protect their less sensitive information. Future CPR systems must implement stricter measures to protect confidentiality (National Research Council, 1991).

Linkages to Secondary Databases

Many clinically relevant registries and databases have evolved in recent years and are of particular interest to health care professionals as they attempt to improve the quality of patient care. Increasingly, these collections of secondary data will be extracted from primary data in CPRs in such a way as to protect the confidentiality and identity of individual patients. Thus, patient records will collect all data on all problems for a single patient; clinical research databases will collect all data on one problem for many patients. For policymakers, the secondary collection of relevant (nonconfidential) clinical information on large populations of patients will support their development of policy strategies and general assessments of quality and outcomes of care. Hundreds of databases are available or are now evolving; some of these resources should be linked with the CPR to provide clinical decision support when needed.

Some current CPR systems already offer linkages to knowledge and research databases. Most CPR systems, however, lack this capacity, owing primarily to the complexity and cost of developing such linkages. Health care professionals are beginning to appreciate the support offered by timely access to a diverse array of external information sources in providing care.

NLM's GRATEFUL MED,[5] for example, gives physicians in their offices ready access to NLM's MEDLINE. For these purposes, it will be important to develop easy-to-use linkages in real time so that feedback to the clinician occurs as part of the decision-making process.

EXPERIENCE WITH CPR SYSTEMS

Health care facilities have been using computers since the 1960s, but that use has primarily focused on business and accounting functions of health care (e.g., patient billing). Many have called these business systems for health care environments either hospital information systems (HISs) or medical information systems (MISs); they have been largely devoid of patient care data. The systems of most interest to this report are clinical information systems, also sometimes known as patient care management systems. Clinical information systems consist of components related to clinical or direct care of patients (Blum, 1986), regardless of the setting (ambulatory, inpatient, institution, or home).

In 1959, two pioneers in health care described a hypothetical health computing system that might be able to address actual clinical problems (Ledley and Lusted, 1960). Almost simultaneously, several other experts began pioneering efforts using computing technologies in clinical settings. By the mid-1960s, Spencer and Vallbona (1965:121) had concluded that at least six areas of medical practice would be affected: "(1) medical diagnosis, (2) hospital medical records, (3) laboratory analysis and functional testing, (4) patient monitoring, (5) hospital communications, and (6) utilization of hospital services and facilities." In 1965, Summerfield and Empey reported that at least 73 hospital and clinical information system projects and 28 projects for storage and retrieval of medical documents and other clinically relevant information were under way. Blum (1984:6) noted that progress through the 1960s was difficult and slow and that "[s]uccesses in information processing during this phase were limited. The Lockheed experience of the late 1960s resulted in the Technicon MIS and a more sobering appraisal of the complexity of clinical information systems."

These early experiences showed that clinical computing offered several distinct challenges that would require significant time to address effectively. A study of clinical systems between 1955 and 1973 by Giebink and

---

[5]GRATEFUL MED is a software tool that runs on a personal computer; it is distributed by the National Library of Medicine. The purpose of GRATEFUL MED is to assist health care professionals and others to search MEDLINE and other databases at the NLM without the assistance of a professional search intermediary. GRATEFUL MED helps the user formulate his or her search query; it also automatically dials and connects to the NLM and then submits the search query to the specified NLM database.

Hurst (1975:xii) revealed that many of the systems planned or developed during the 1960s were "extinct—blunt testimony to the difficulties of implementing computer based information systems for health care delivery. . . . Medical computer applications which meet operational criteria are rare except for routine business applications. . . . Other than in developmental projects, computerized medical records are abstracts of more complete records maintained in hard copy form."

With the advent of less costly mini- and microcomputers, clinical information system development flourished during the 1970s and 1980s. The advances made during these years focused primarily on departmental systems (known today as subsystems) for such areas as the clinical laboratory, radiology, electrocardiology, and the pharmacy. One reason for this flurry of development was that departmental systems were easier and less risky to develop than comprehensive systems covering patient care management.

The 1970s and 1980s also saw the development of systems for clinical decision support (Warner et al., 1972; Shortliffe, 1987). To perform their sophisticated functions, these complex systems require that at least a subset of the CPR be available as input—that is, in machine-readable form. Once the use of CPRs becomes more widespread and more and more patient data are captured, these systems should become increasingly valuable to clinicians.

Virtually all of the current clinical information systems that might qualify as CPR systems have evolved from a strong academic medical center's teaching hospital or clinic records. Examples of this phenomenon include the COSTAR[6] (Computer Stored Ambulatory Record; Barnett, 1984) system, which is used by several institutions, including the Harvard Community Health Plan; a system used by the Latter-Day Saints Hospital in Salt Lake City, Utah, known as Health Evaluation through Logical Processing (HELP),[7] which was developed by faculty at the University of Utah (Warner et al., 1972; Pryor et al., 1983, 1984); the TMR (The Medical Record) system at Duke University Medical Center (Stead and Hammond, 1988); and the THERESA system at Grady Memorial Hospital, the primary teaching hospital for Emory University's medical school (Walker, 1989).

With few exceptions, software developed in an academic setting is not generally considered to be particularly robust or of an "industrial or commercial grade"; consequently, some experts have been skeptical about the functionality of these and other clinical information systems. Nevertheless, many of these systems have proved their usefulness and viability in supporting the actual delivery of health care in real-world settings. Attributes

---

[6]COSTAR is a registered trademark of Massachusetts General Hospital.
[7]HELP is a registered trademark of 3M.

of the systems discussed above are presented in subsequent sections of this chapter.

These systems all illustrate the time required to establish operational clinical systems: all of them began development at least a decade ago, and some have been under development for more than two decades. Now, however, their increasingly sophisticated capabilities are being recognized in the marketplace. A variety of commercial organizations, having seen or demonstrated the viability of these systems in one or more hospital or clinic settings, have subsequently negotiated further developmental and marketing rights to these clinical information systems.

AN OVERVIEW OF CPR SYSTEMS

A distinguishing feature of the clinical information systems that can rightly be called computer-based patient record systems is their underlying database management system. Generally, for performance reasons, CPR systems have developed their own DBMS and have avoided the use of commercially available products. As a result, they use an approach by which a data dictionary can be expanded to accommodate new data elements to be captured in the CPR. Such flexibility sets these systems apart for two reasons: (1) their databases are not fixed in terms of size and content, and (2) no significant reprogramming is needed to meet the continually changing demands placed on the CPR system by technology innovations and system enhancements.

Much of the effort to automate clinical functions has focused on a single department such as the laboratory or pharmacy; these are not examples of CPR systems. The more noteworthy examples of currently operating CPR systems go well beyond the routine collection, storage, and communication of data provided by one or more departmental systems. Yet, to reiterate, no single health care information system operational in 1990 captures and manipulates the entire CPR. Of those that might qualify as CPR systems, not one is comprehensive enough to serve as a model for the future computer-based systems that will be designed to manage the entire patient care record.

The few clinical information systems that qualify as "today's CPR systems" share several common traits. First, they maintain a large data dictionary to define the contents of their internal CPRs. Second, all patient data recorded in the CPR are tagged with the time and date of the transaction, thus making the CPR a continuous chronological history of the patient's medical care. Third, the systems retrieve and report data in the CPR in a flexible manner. Finally, the systems offer a research tool for using the CPR data.

Although much remains to be done to design and produce complete, robust CPR systems, significant progress has been made in establishing state-of-the-art components of CPR systems. Several systems developed in recent years have been designed and tailored to serve the special needs of nearly all members of the health care team in a variety of health care settings.

This section discusses a few key attributes of selected operational clinical systems that effectively utilize some portion of a computer-based patient record. There has been no attempt to provide an exhaustive presentation here of all the clinical systems developed to date. Rather, the discussion below focuses on systems that embody one or more special features crucial to the successful implementation of the complete CPR, especially within certain practice settings. These include (1) physician offices and group practice settings, (2) health maintenance organizations, (3) single hospitals or medical centers, and (4) large multihospital systems. By a large margin, the majority of patient care is provided in the office or group practice setting; as a result, systems that specifically address the needs of practitioners and patients in this environment will probably encounter the most substantial challenges and have the greatest impact. Therefore, although only two systems in this category are discussed below (many others have been developed or are currently under development), it should be understood that this category comprises perhaps the most important settings for CPR systems in terms of the potential for improved care. In addition to the discussion of clinical systems, the section also describes a few international developments of special interest and selected emerging developments.

Physician Offices and Group Practice Settings

The Medical Record

For more than 20 years, the Duke University Medical Center[8] has been developing a comprehensive medical information system known as The Medical Record (TMR). The TMR system was first conceived as a tool for clinicians in outpatient settings; it was subsequently expanded to address the needs of clinicians in inpatient settings (Hammond and Stead, 1986). From the outset of the project, the CPR was considered the centerpiece of the TMR system (Stead and Hammond, 1988). The system can store and retrieve any data contained in a traditional paper record in an ambulatory or inpatient setting, with the exception of images such as X-rays. In an inpa-

---

[8]William E. Hammond of Duke University Medical Center supplied the explanation and description of the TMR system. Where possible, the information was checked for consistency with published articles in peer-reviewed journals. The Medical Record and TMR are registered trademarks of Database, Inc.

tient setting, however, the TMR system can provide a link to such imaging systems.

The TMR system can support a complete list of diagnoses and procedures, as well as subjective and physical findings, laboratory data, and therapeutic interventions. The system also allows multiple "views" of data. For example, patient data may be viewed from any of several perspectives—from a problem, time, task, or encounter orientation.[9] The look and feel of a particular TMR system are controlled by a user-defined, object-oriented data dictionary that separates the parameters, or variables, along which data are being collected from the system features that manipulate those variables. Even users with no programming expertise thus can tailor the TMR to their own needs.

Health Maintenance Organizations

Computer-Stored Ambulatory Record Systems

In 1968 the Laboratory of Computer Science at the Massachusetts General Hospital implemented the COSTAR (Computer Stored Ambulatory Record) system, which became one of the first systems capable of producing a computer-based patient record.[10] COSTAR is a medical information management and record system designed as a set of modules for which individual sites can choose the portions of the system they wish to install. COSTAR supports patient registration, scheduling of patient visits, storage and retrieval of clinical information, and billing and accounts receivable (Barnett, 1984).

---

[9]Patient records and the optimal formats for organizing and presenting their data have been under discussion for more than 20 years (Weed, 1968). There are four major types of approaches for organizing and presenting clinical data in a patient record. The *problem-oriented record* links the patient's clinical data with his or her problems so that all aspects of the care process are focused on resolving those problems. The *time-oriented view* of the patient's clinical data is more organizational than philosophical. Entries in the record appear in chronological sequence, reflecting what was decided upon and what was done at specific times. *Task-oriented records* emphasize the tasks undertaken to care for the patient and present the patient's care organized in ways specific to those who routinely perform certain sets of tasks. The *encounter-oriented record* is an organized view of the patient's care processes structured by the encounters of the patient (often over a long period of time). An encounter is defined as a hospital stay or treatment for a single problem, regardless of how long the treatment may last (sometimes years).

[10]G. Octo Barnett, Harvard Medical School, provided the general description of COSTAR. Where possible, reference is also made to published articles in peer-reviewed journals. Stephen G. Schoenbaum, also affiliated with Harvard Medical School, provided the explanation and description of the COSTAR system at the Harvard Community Health Plan.

The first implementation of COSTAR was at the Harvard Community Health Plan (HCHP), which adopted and began testing the COSTAR systems in 1969 (Grossman et al., 1973). By 1987, HCHP had installed 10 minicomputers to support clinical computing in their 9 care facilities, which together serve an active membership of more than 225,000 people. The HCHP COSTAR system now contains individual records for nearly 550,000 people generated over the past 20 years.

The HCHP system supports patient record inquiry, a tumor registry, clinical reminders, and storage and retrieval of demographic data. It also provides clinical reporting, automated appointment scheduling, and diverse management reports and facilitates urgent care. Much of the patient record can be printed on demand by clinicians, and by 1986 more than 4.1 million pages were being printed annually (Harvard Community Health Plan, n.d.). In that same year 1.3 million patient encounters were documented, more than 2.5 million lines of text were dictated and transcribed into the system, and the results of 650,000 laboratory tests were entered.

Two characteristics of COSTAR have made it possible to use the system in a variety of sites. One is modular design: a site need only install a partial set of modules—for example, scheduling and medical record modules but not the accounting module. The other is its substantial, extensible data dictionary. The core of the data dictionary is a controlled vocabulary of clinical terms, which includes the ability to associate modifier terms with the primary name for a clinical concept. These modifiers make the COSTAR controlled vocabulary quite sophisticated: it can provide synonyms and generate specialized terms by combining the modifier with the primary name for a concept. It can also associate specific brand names with the generic names for drugs.

The COSTAR system is comprehensive enough to include all major categories of clinical data, including laboratory results and findings from diagnostic procedures. All data recorded in the patient record are associated with controlled vocabulary terms (and any selected modifiers). The benefits of this approach are seen in clinical care (e.g., for any patient, the system can generate a summary document that contains the most recent information on every COSTAR code in the record); quality assurance (e.g., the system can analyze each patient record to identify patients with certain risk factors for whom an influenza vaccination is indicated); and clinical investigation (e.g., the system can examine the patterns of prescription ordering for hypertension by physicians with different levels of training).

In 1975 the Laboratory of Computer Science rewrote the system and made it available in the public domain. Currently, there is an active COSTAR users' group that provides information about the system, conducts tutorials, and distributes COSTAR manuals and software on diskettes for a nominal fee. A number of commercial vendors also market COSTAR. Current system users of COSTAR include physician offices, public health departments, ambulatory care clinics, a veterinary teaching clinic, and a consortium of sites for multiple sclerosis research. COSTAR has been implemented in several hundred sites in the United States, Canada, Mexico, Argentina, and Europe.

Single Hospitals or Medical Centers

THERESA System

Atlanta's Grady Memorial Hospital, the primary clinical teaching facility of the Emory University School of Medicine, contracted with Medical Systems Development for the development of its CPR system in 1981. As of 1990 there were 18 million documents on-line. Plans call for completing the system in late 1991, illustrating again the complexity and length of time required to create an operational clinical system.

THERESA,[11] as Grady's system is called, is based on a custom-made, object-oriented database management system that was specially designed to address the problems associated with the patient record noted earlier in this report (see Chapter 2). It supports problem-oriented, task-oriented, event-oriented, and time-oriented "views" of the patient record. It also permits users to employ English-like queries to access the complete database. When a user requests complex decision support, the system searches the database, typically requiring from 30 seconds to 3 minutes to respond to the user's request. Since the first modules became operational at Grady in 1983, data on more than 220,000 patient encounters (an encounter is defined as a single hospital stay or clinic visit) have been collected; the patient record includes data on the individual's medical history, physical examination, and diagnosis, as well as orders, results, progress notes, and physician and nursing notes. The system maintains a lifelong record and never deletes clinical data.

Physicians and other members of the health care team enter these data directly using "windowing" terminals (a feature that permits users to look at different data or views of the same data on the terminal screen at the same time). The majority of data are entered using a mouse (i.e., point-and-click technology; Walker, 1989). A recent analysis of one month's medical admissions revealed that practitioners entered complete data on 98 percent of

---

[11]Kenneth Walker of the Emory University School of Medicine supplied the explanation and description of this system. The committee attempted to check the information for consistency with published articles concerning the system in peer-reviewed journals but was unable to locate any such reports. However, other information in such journals supports the description given here.

their patients. THERESA is therefore one of the few clinical systems that have successfully engaged clinicians in direct patient data entry. Grady also appears to have successfully solved the problem of ensuring system access. Although it has not installed expensive special fault-tolerant computer systems,[12] for the last seven years a distributed network of standard supermini-computers has provided access to the system 99.95 percent of the time.

Health Evaluation Through Logical Processing

The Intermountain Health Care Corporation's Latter-Day Saints (LDS) Hospital provides another example of the CPR system of today.[13] The LDS system, which has been under development for more than 25 years, is known as HELP (Health Evaluation through Logical Processing; Pryor et al., 1983). HELP's primary objective is to provide medical decision support, but it is also a computer-based patient record system. Much of the input to HELP comes directly from medical professionals entering data at terminals, but wherever possible HELP utilizes automated input of the patient's clinical data. Although LDS has conducted experiments using an automated patient history, currently only minimal history and physical examination data are contained in the HELP record. Consequently, at present, HELP maintains both a paper and a computer-based record for each patient.

Developers of HELP have consistently tried to focus on the use of patient data in making decisions about care rather than on merely the storage and communication of these data. To support its decision-making goals, HELP contains more than 100,000 rules and statistical processes pertaining to a broad spectrum of health care; it uses these rules and processes to make decisions (including diagnoses)—just as a panel of experts might when presented with similar data. The system makes decisions in both a background monitoring mode and an interactive session with the health care

---

[12]Fault-tolerant computer systems have been developed by the computer industry to provide virtually uninterrupted service to users. To achieve such an objective, these systems offer a high degree of component redundancy in the hardware as well as sensors and special additional rerouting components. If embedded sensors detect that a crucial system component has failed, the system automatically switches to a redundant component to maintain continuous service. Although such systems are costly, they have in recent years become the mainstay for support of an organization's essential applications. Therefore, fault-tolerant computer systems are often of particular interest to CPR system vendors and developers.

[13]T. Allan Pryor of the University of Utah Department of Medical Informatics supplied the explanation and description of this system. Where possible, the information was checked for consistency with published articles in peer-reviewed journals.

provider. To maintain constant availability of the system, HELP has been developed to run on special fault-tolerant computers.

Beth Israel and Brigham and Women's Hospital System

The clinical information system at Beth Israel Hospital in Boston, Massachusetts, was developed by the Harvard Medical School's Center for Clinical Computing and has been in continuous use and evolution for more than a decade (Bleich and Slack, 1989).[14] The system at Brigham and Women's Hospital in Boston, also from the Clinical Computing Center, was modeled after Beth Israel's system and required approximately four years to develop. More than 800 and more than 1,250 on-line terminals currently operate at Beth Israel and Brigham and Women's hospitals, respectively (Safran et al., 1989). One outstanding attribute of these systems is their extensive use by clinicians and other members of the health care team. At Beth Israel during an average week, for example, 742 departmental and laboratory workers entered or corrected information in computer-based patient records 137,526 times (Bleich et al., 1989). Similarly, during an average week, 532 physicians, 893 nurses, 59 medical students, and 253 health assistants used the computer terminals to examine patient information.

In addition to reporting results, these systems provide other capabilities to clinicians: scheduling, order entry, electronic mail, and bibliographic retrieval through PaperChase. Beth Israel users can also search the growing clinical database. This retrieval capability, called ClinQuery (Safran et al., 1989), is a powerful tool for answering administrative and research questions. Through this system, hospital practitioners can access the *Physicians' Desk Reference* (PDR) and receive advice from an attached expert system designed to assist practitioners in treating acid-base problems.

Clinical computing systems at these two hospitals are patient centered and integrated rather than networked or interfaced (i.e., they utilize the central database model displayed in Figure 3-1). These systems also store data for hospitalized and ambulatory patients in a common database within each institution. In addition, the systems handle patient billing functions. Indeed, installation of these clinical computing systems has reduced substantially the length of time between provision of service and receipt of payment for the service. (Accounts receivable dropped by 30 days at Beth Israel when the clinical computing system was installed; when that system

---

[14]Warner V. Slack and Charles Safran of the Center for Clinical Computing at Harvard supplied the explanation and description of this system. Where possible, the information was checked for consistency with published articles in peer-reviewed journals.

also performed the fiscal computing, accounts receivable dropped by 40 days.) The experience of Beth Israel and Brigham and Women's hospitals shows that clinical computer systems can drive nearly all patient billing functions and that they can do so more efficiently than separate machines dedicated only to patient billing. Slack (1989:140) notes that "more than 90% of each patient's charges are now collected as a byproduct of the clinical computing system." This important feature substantiates the dual notions that the CPR is or should be the central feature of all clinical systems and that it is capable of supporting nearly every functional component of the system, including billing.

Lockheed's Early Clinical Information System

One of the earliest demonstrations of a clinical information system came through the development of a system by the Lockheed Corporation between the mid-1960s and 1970s. Technicon, an early clinical system vendor, acquired the system from Lockheed; today, it is owned and marketed by a company called TDS. This system displays two distinct, powerful features crucial to the design of future CPR systems. First, it offers very fast response times (usually less than one second) for nearly all user input; second, it is extremely flexible. For example, it can support the diverse needs of many users at a single site because the system has been tailored to meet the expectations of several simultaneous users.

Large Multihospital Systems

Department of Veterans Affairs

A pioneer and leader in this field, the Department of Veterans Affairs (VA) has been developing its clinical computing system, known as the Decentralized Hospital Computer Program (DHCP), for nearly a decade (Andrews and Beauchamp, 1989). By the late 1980s, the VA had installed DHCP in most of its more than 170 medical centers.[15] Outpatient clinics and other care facilities, including nursing homes, operated by the VA gain access to systems through the VA's national network.

The VA's DHCP consists of software grouped into three categories: (1)

---

[15]At the direction of Congress the VA has installed commercially developed clinical information systems in a few selected VA medical centers to test the VA's DHCP against systems from the private sector. All other VA medical centers have installed and are using the DHCP. All of the VA's medical centers thus use automated clinical systems—that is, one or the other of these two approaches.

system/database management, (2) administrative management, and (3) clinical management. System/database management software consists of software tools that have been constructed by the VA for the support, development, and maintenance of the DHCP. Administrative management software supports all normal hospital administrative tasks, including scheduling. Clinical management software supports clinical information provision in the laboratory, pharmacy, and other departments. It includes a complete surgery module and also partially supports medicine, cardiology, and oncology. The VA is recognized for its use of state-of-the-art technologies in selected radiology departments (Dayhoff et al., 1990).

To advance the clinical aspects of the DHCP, the VA has launched the Clinical Record Project. Clinical record development is under way at several sites and includes modules to support order entry/results reporting, a health summary, a problem index, allergies/adverse reactions, progress notes, crisis warnings, consults information, clinical observations, and clinical measurements. These and other clinical modules represent the VA's commitment to constructing its own state-of-the-art CPR system.

Department of Defense

The Department of Defense (DoD) has contracted for the deployment of a clinical information system at its hundreds of care facilities around the world (General Accounting Office [GAO], 1988, 1990). The system, known as the Composite Health Care System (CHCS), is currently being tested in multiple care facilities in the United States that serve a range of care settings. One example involves health maintenance organization-like settings in Hawaii where hospitals and associated care facilities and clinics are networked. As military personnel visit any of these facilities, the CHCS allows clinicians to gain immediate access to patient care data from previous patient encounters.

The CHCS is an excellent environment and opportunity to design, test, and evaluate certain desirable features of the ideal CPR system, and its potential in this regard may prove vital to accelerating the development of CPR systems generally. For example, the military has established a command structure that permits testing in a closed-loop environment. This means that, within limits, DoD can mandate particular clinician behaviors to evaluate various potentially beneficial methods of providing care and that the CHCS can measure the benefits, if any, that are derived. Currently, the CHCS represents the largest demonstration of actual clinician hands-on data entry to clinical systems: because military facility commanders can require clinicians to input data into the system, alternative input mechanisms may be evaluated. In addition, DoD is testing a prototype professional workstation to facilitate clinicians' interaction with the CHCS.

International Developments

DIOGENE

DIOGENE, a system operating in the largest hospital in Geneva, Switzer-land, supports a nearly complete CPR and will soon support communication of high-resolution images throughout the hospital complex. The system's unique approach to clinical data capture (Scherrer et al., 1990) may well offer a useful model that could be utilized in other health care organizations.

DIOGENE employs specially trained transcriptionists who can enter text rapidly. A clinician who wants to enter narrative into the patient's computer-based record first identifies or displays the record on a computer terminal near the point of care. He or she then places a call to an available transcriptionist on a nearby telephone and begins dictating. As the dictation proceeds, the typed narrative appears on the terminal display currently being used by the clinician. At the completion of the dictation the clinician suggests any pertinent changes and then approves the text, which becomes a permanent part of the computer-based patient record in DIOGENE.

Even at peak hours, a few specially trained transcriptionists can support all practitioners' dictation. In the future, when clinical workstations can accept direct voice input, transcriptionists will no longer be required.

The Exmouth Project

A large experimental study, known as the Exmouth Project, is being conducted in Exeter, England. The experiment uses patient-carried "smart cards"[16] capable of storing critical portions of the complete patient record that are essential in emergency as well as routine care situations. In Exeter, 98 percent of the pharmacies, 70 percent of general practitioners, and all hospitals are able to read and use the credit card-sized patient Care Cards.

---

[16]Smart cards are electronic devices (usually encased in plastic) that resemble a credit card one might carry in a wallet. To date, these cards are more popular in Europe than elsewhere and are used in a variety of applications, from banking and financial transactions to medical applications. They contain electronic circuitry capable of storing limited amounts of information crucial to the specific application for which the card is intended. For example, in a health care application, a patient's card might ideally contain such things as demographic information, payer information, allergy history, blood type, personal and family history, environmental and other risk factors, a photograph of the patient, a record of the last 10 vital sign readings (perhaps revealing trends such as hypertension), current medications, recent but former medications, discharge summaries from the last three hospitalizations, and other information that might prove vital in providing health care, especially in an emergency situation. Similar to drivers' licenses the card would be carried at all times. When the patient appeared for care or in an emergency situation, the card could be made available to all members of the health care team.

This experiment is driven by the belief that information management in health care is a primary key to cost containment. Approximately 9,000 patient Care Cards (which includes cards for all diabetics in the area) are in routine use. Preliminary results of the test released in late 1990 reveal significant reductions in staff time devoted to clerical functions, a significant increase in patient-centered activities by clinicians, and significant reductions in orders for laboratory tests (presumably because recent test results were available from the Care Card). Patients themselves indicated significantly greater satisfaction with the care they have received since introduction of the cards in 1989 (only 2 percent expressed dissatisfaction; Hopkins, 1990).

England has also embarked on a large experiment in which more than 16,000 general practitioners have installed personal computers in their offices to support clinical practice. This figure represents approximately half of all general practitioners in the country and is perhaps the most substantial (in terms of numbers of practitioners) clinical computing experiment undertaken to date. These and other experiments in Europe imply that Europeans have significant experience in developing clinical data standards, perhaps more than most other regions of the world. Further, they indicate the very real need for greater international cooperation in formulating future health care data standards.

Selected Emerging Developments

Once a patient's clinical data are in machine-readable form, many decision-making aids will be available to health care professionals to permit them to take advantage of the latest information on problems specific to the patient. In addition, clinical data in the CPR may support other capabilities that can help ensure higher quality care, one beneficial consequence of which may be a reduction in the rate of malpractice suits. Several of these recently developed decision-making aids are described below.

Chart Checker

Kaufman and Holbrook (1990) describe Chart Checker, a software package that operates in conjunction with the machine-readable emergency room record. Chart Checker analyzes the emergency room record narrative to alert the emergency room physician to potentially serious diagnoses that he or she may have overlooked or dismissed too quickly. This capability is particularly important for preventing malpractice suits. For example, Kaufman and Holbrook (1990) noted that more than 30 percent of liability cases won against emergency room physicians resulted from missing a myocardial infarction. Chart Checker has been tested using emergency room narratives for cases in which myocardial infarctions actually occurred, and the package quite accurately suggested the possibility of that diagnosis, as well as other potentially devastating illnesses that apparently had not been seriously considered.

Chart Checker's benefits are so well demonstrated that in certain instances it has led to an across-the-board 20 percent reduction in malpractice insurance premiums for physicians. In Massachusetts, for example, this reduction in premiums (amounting to $2,400 or more per physician) became effective in July 1990 for all emergency room physicians who regularly use Chart Checker (Blau, 1990). This software is representative of many clinical decision support systems that can be expected to evolve in the near future. Such tools cannot be used by health care professionals, however, until clinical data are captured in machine-readable form. In short, the CPR must come first.

Problem-Knowledge Coupler

The problem-knowledge coupler (PKC) is another personal computer-based system designed to assist clinicians in organizing patient data in a variety of care settings (Weed, in press). Weed's system permits the clinician to build a computer-based, problem-oriented patient record; it also uses medical knowledge derived from the literature to provide the clinician with timely suggestions and information specific to the symptoms or problems of the current patient to guide and assist the clinician's decision making. Thus, the PKC presents a nearly complete list of potential causes of a patient's reported problems. Only a few topics in medicine have been covered so far, however, because many couplers have yet to be written.

The PKC is designed to provide practitioners with information they need from the literature when they need it. At the moment, the system supplies references to highly relevant, targeted articles that have been searched beforehand and are directly associated with the patient's problems. Some of the system's architects have proposed that a ready link to MEDLINE at the NLM is the solution to answering clinicians' questions near the time of the patient encounter. Currently, however, that notion may be unrealistic because the time required to formulate and perform an adequate bibliographic search is measured in minutes, not seconds.

Medical Logic Modules

Decision support systems for health care have been successfully demonstrated in recent years, but they too lack a common standard for representing the knowledge they contain, thus limiting exchanges of their contents (Pryor et al., 1984; Miller et al., 1986). As special medical knowledge databases are developed at different institutions, the ability to share these data-bases will become important. Anticipating this need, the Center for Medical Informatics at the Columbia Presbyterian Medical Center has been exploring and testing the development of the Arden syntax for medical logic modules (Hripcsak et al., 1990). The Arden syntax is designed to facilitate the sharing of medical knowledge and is especially well suited for the transfer of medical knowledge bases among disparate medical decision support systems.

Clinical data derived from operational CPR systems will contribute significantly to the body of medical knowledge used by future medical decision support systems. Indeed, it is highly probable that CPR systems may realize their full impact only when used in conjunction with medical decision support systems. Similarly, medical decision support systems are likely to mature only when medical knowledge can be readily transferred between systems. Therefore, indirectly, the Arden syntax may be crucial to the rate of CPR system deployment.

CLINICIAN INTERACTION AND RESISTANCE

Perhaps the single greatest challenge that has consistently confronted every clinical system developer is to engage clinicians in direct data entry. Clinical systems have used many different strategies to solve this problem; they range from eliminating the need for clinician input to mandating direct data entry by clinicians.

The LDS Hospital in Salt Lake City, Utah, is a good example of an innovative approach to circumvent resistance to clinician data entry. As discussed earlier in this chapter, the hospital's HELP system directly captures clinical data (from the laboratory, intensive care units, and other departments) virtually without human intervention wherever possible; it uses specially designed data-capture devices attached to conventional medical instruments that convert analog to digital information. Today, most vendors of such medical instruments and devices provide computer-ready output capabilities as standard equipment or as options.

Other systems require data to be typed by clinicians or by some intermediary. Yet the bulk of the patient record is still unstructured text, such as the patient history, the discharge summary, and physical examination findings; this text must be entered into the clinical system either by dictation, which must be transcribed in some timely manner, or by automated speech-recognition systems. Another alternative is for the information to be typed manually into the system. Many system developers have attempted to use typed input, but this approach has generally failed because busy clinicians reject it. The next section discusses possible technical support to overcome clinician resistance to interacting with CPR systems.

Finding appropriate mechanisms to encourage direct clinician input remains a significant challenge for clinical system architects (Mandell, 1987; Benda, 1989). Experience demonstrates that providing a fee for data entry does have a positive impact. For example, the New England Deaconess Hospital found in an initial test in 1989 that paying $5 to physicians to input their own discharge summaries directly resulted in a 40 percent participation rate. Without escalating payment, 54 percent of the discharge summaries (in some months, as many as 70 percent) were entered into the system directly by physicians during the first six months of 1990 (Zibrak et al., 1990).

TECHNOLOGICAL BARRIERS

Several technological barriers still must be overcome before robust CPR systems can be fully realized, although no great technological breakthroughs are needed. The human interface—the place where man and machine meet— remains a major challenge (despite such advances as the graphical user interface and voice inputting) and is closely tied to system performance. As we move further into the 1990s, the major technological barriers to widespread implementation of the CPR include problems with text processing, the lack of appropriate confidentiality or security measures, and inadequate health data-exchange standards.

The Human Interface and System Performance

The lack of sufficiently powerful computing systems at an affordable price has been a major barrier to providing clinicians with an adequate human interface. Now, however, affordable state-of-the-art computer systems have been introduced, which are likely to resolve this problem. Slack (1989) argues that users of clinical systems require a response time of less than a second. Providing a simple-to-use, or nearly intuitive, human interface means dedicating a significant proportion of the computer's resources to that function, which reduces their availability for crucial clinical functions. As a result, clinical system architects in the past have generally been inclined to emphasize clinical function and performance at the expense of the human interface.

The most natural way for humans to communicate is through speech, and a great deal of computer science research has focused for decades on voice-recognition capabilities. Recently introduced, commercially viable systems address this problem in ways that are becoming acceptable to some in the health care sector, but currently available, affordable voice-recognition systems support only a portion of the health care requirements.

Three primary criteria must be met to enable widespread, effective use of such systems. First, the ability to accept and process continuous speech, that is, speaking without pausing between each individual word, is crucial.

Second, systems should be speaker independent; that is, the system should be able to recognize words spoken by any individual who might speak without first "training" the system to recognize the words spoken by that individual. Third, systems for general medicine require large vocabularies; some domains and subdomains, for example, may require vocabularies in excess of 30,000 words or meaningful phrases. As vocabularies expand, both the costs and error rates generally become intolerable. Emerging voice-recognition technology is likely to ease the inputting of clinical data in future CPR systems, but the successful experiences discussed earlier with such systems as HELP, THERESA, and DIOGENE confirm the existence of currently available alternative approaches to capturing crucial clinical data (including text) in the CPR.

Text Processing

Assuming that text can be conveniently entered into the clinical system through voice-recognition technology or other means, the problem then becomes one of effectively analyzing in an automated way the content and meaning of the textual data. The raw material for epidemiological analysis and for effectiveness and outcomes studies is primarily text from patient records, which must be converted to coded data. For accurate comparisons, patient record data must be correctly transformed into precise, unambiguous codes that represent specific characteristic processes.

Text processing is generally considered to be a complex operation; its application to the data in the CPR, with its special and diverse vocabularies, further complicates the challenge of implementing it as a system capability. Often, the more experienced the practitioner, the more succinct or abbreviated the notes in the record. The notes thus may consist of abbreviations, acronyms, and mnemonics, which could be difficult to interpret, even by other health care professionals. Although text processors have improved markedly in recent years, they can approach but never exceed the quality of written or dictated information. Therefore, the quality of patient records can be improved only through more disciplined approaches to consistent vocabulary in the record. Although technology (voice-input or menu-driven input systems) can artificially impose more consistent terminology, practitioners should be encouraged as a rule to avoid idiosyncratic terminology and to use more formal, well-defined vocabularies. Additional technological research is needed in this area, as well as studies of incentives for behavioral change, before CPR systems can reach their full potential.

Confidentiality and Security

Among the important priorities for the 1990s is the further development

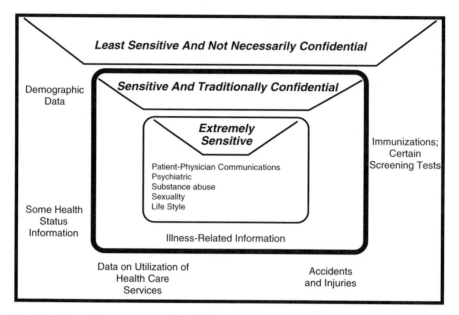

FIGURE 3.2   Three-zone confidentiality model.

of technology to ensure fully the privacy and confidentiality of patient data in the CPR. Indeed, as discussed in Chapter 4, societal and legal concerns about privacy and confidentiality must be satisfactorily resolved before wide-scale implementation of the CPR can occur. Many technologies are available to ensure CPR security and integrity, but, in general, they have not been adequately deployed or embedded in present CPR systems.

Recent research has proposed a three-zone medical confidentiality model (Figure 3-2). In this model, extremely sensitive information, which would always be held confidential, resides in the innermost zone and might not always find its way into the CPR. The outermost zone contains the least sensitive information, which may or may not be confidential. The area between these two zones is the one containing sensitive information, probably related mainly to illnesses and health problems; it is likely to be the largest area in terms of volume of the CPR and the one most frequently associated with traditional medical confidentiality requirements.

The figure illustrates why CPR systems must address confidentiality adequately at multiple levels. Patients should be permitted to name the portions of their record that are to remain totally confidential (i.e., the innermost information zone). Practitioners may also designate elements of the CPR as highly confidential. Most of the emphasis on confidentiality has involved protecting patient-related information in the CPR, but confidentiality issues may also pertain to others engaged in providing health care. For example, all members of the health care team deserve the same level of protection against unauthorized access or abuse of information in the CPR that applies to the patient.

One important method for ensuring confidentiality, and data and program integrity, is to allow access to the CPR system only to those with a need to know and then to certify positively their identity before granting access. Fortunately, the problem of implementing measures to ensure confidentiality and privacy is not unique to medicine. Confidentiality issues are important in several areas outside health care such as finance and banking, libraries, and communications, and these sectors may offer approaches that could be tailored to the needs of health care users. For example, future CPR systems must be capable of providing different levels of data confidentiality as required by their users. Psychiatric data are a case in point: they must be available only to the patient's psychiatrist. In addition, some sensitive data for drug abuse, alcoholism, and similarly sensitive diagnoses must be protected by legal and professional rules and regulations.

Health Data-Exchange Standards

Progress toward developing acceptable standards for transferring an entire CPR has been slow, primarily because standards development has been largely ad hoc. Still, although such progress is meager in comparison to what is needed, it appears impressive when one considers that it has been accomplished virtually without government funding and without substantial industry-wide commitment. Nevertheless, the lack of funding for and coordination of standards development for CPRs can constitute a major barrier to CPR development, testing, and deployment. What is perhaps of even greater concern, given the current limited support for standards development, is the potential long-term negative impact of premature standards development. Without substantially better coordination and greater funding relatively soon, standards may evolve that may later prove to be inadequate, and neither as well conceived nor as robust as the standards needed to support a broad array of future CPR applications.

Before an actual exchange of clinical data can take place, agreement must be reached on what is being transferred. Many vendors and government agencies have independently developed their own internal clinical data dictionaries. These dictionaries differ in terms of the actual data elements included, naming conventions, definitions, and relationships among data elements. No attempt has yet been made to create a composite clinical data dictionary (CCDD) using input provided by these and other groups interested in the CPR (Figure 3-3). For example, the federal government alone has at least three distinct clinical data dictionaries (namely, those of DoD, the VA, and the Health Care

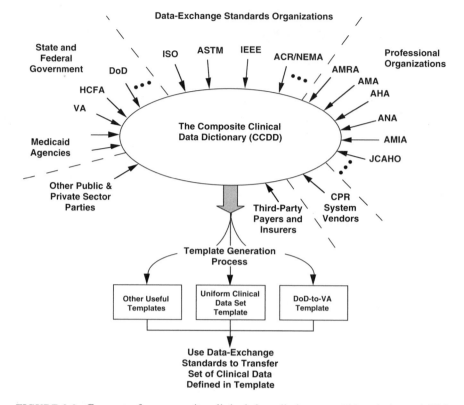

FIGURE 3-3 Concept of a composite clinical data dictionary. Abbreviations: ACR/ NEMA, American College of Radiologists/National Electrical Manufacturers Association; AHA, American Hospital Association; AMA, American Medical Association; AMIA, American Medical Informatics Association; AMRA, American Medical Record Association; ANA, American Nurses Association; ASTM, American Society for Testing Materials; DoD, Department of Defense; HCFA, Health Care Financing Administration; IEEE, Institute of Electronic and Electrical Engineers; ISO, International Standards Organization; JCAHO, Joint Commission on Accreditation of Healthcare Organizations; VA, Department of Veterans Affairs.

Financing Administration); each of these has evolved independently and largely without coordination. Because no CCDD yet exists, the evolution of data-exchange standards has been limited and will remain so until a CCDD or some similar coordinating mechanism is developed.

Once a CCDD is created and perpetually maintained, any number of relevant subsets can be generated from this defined universe of clinical content. Standard definitions of subsets (or "templates," as shown in Figure 3-3) can be prepared, and data-exchange standards can then be used to carry out the actual data transfers. For example, one potential template might be HCFA's Uniform Clinical Data Set (UCDS), a collection of approximately 1,600 data elements (Krakauer, 1990). Over time, many other relevant data sets for varied purposes are likely to be generated using subsets from the universe of data elements defined in the CCDD. For example, emergency room (ER) physicians might designate a small set of clinical data elements from the CCDD (such a subset could be the ER template) that are required to facilitate appropriate care in an emergency setting. This template could then be used to formulate an appropriate health data-exchange standard to perform the actual transfer of patient data between disparate CPR systems.

The diversity of patient record data is likely to continue as a number of different vendors and mix of institutions, service bureaus, reimbursement agencies, and governmental agencies increase their use of clinical data. It is essential, therefore, that development and promotion of standards for data representation and data exchange be major priorities. Without such standards, it will be impossible to support the necessary exchange of CPR data among the different interested organizations and institutions.

SUMMARY

Although progress has been steady over the past two decades in developing complete CPR systems, and although several powerful clinical information systems have become operational in recent years, as yet not one is capable of supporting the complete CPR. Most of the former technological barriers to developing CPR systems have now or are about to disappear, and no technological breakthroughs are needed to implement CPR systems. Nevertheless, further maturation of a few emerging technologies, such as voice-input or voice-recognition and text-processing systems, would facilitate the development of state-of-the-art CPR systems in the 1990s.

Many different standards must be developed, tested, and deployed before the CPR can realize its full potential. Standards to facilitate the exchange of health care data are needed now so that clinical data may be aggregated and analyzed to support improved decision making. When clinical data from CPR systems are pooled in regional and national databases and made available through networks, they will constitute a vast information resource on which to base health care policy, clinical studies of effectiveness and appropriateness, and equitable reimbursement policies.

Standards are also needed for the development of more secure CPR systems. All of this effort should focus on ensuring the integrity of the clinical data in the CPR and on patient confidentiality. Confidentiality of health data in CPR systems is crucial to the success of these systems. Further, confidentiality must be maintained not only for the patient but for all health care professionals and especially for members of the health care team.

Although powerful new technologies and standards will greatly facilitate the realization of the CPR, they alone are not sufficient to overcome the barriers to its routine use. The primary barriers to realizing complete CPR systems are not technical but rather behavioral or organizational in nature. The next chapter explores various means for overcoming such barriers.

REFERENCES

Andrews, R. D., and C. Beauchamp. 1989. A clinical database management system for improved integration of the Veterans Affairs hospital information system. *Journal of Medical Systems* 13:309-320.

ASTM (American Society for Testing Materials). 1989. *Standard Guide for Nosologic Standards and Guides for Construction of New Biomedical Nomenclature.* Report No. E 1284-89. Philadelphia, Pa.

Barnett, G. O. 1984. The application of computer based medical record systems in ambulatory care. *New England Journal of Medicine* 310:1643-1650.

Barnett, G. O., R. Zielstorff, J. Piggins, M. McLatchey, M. Morgan, S. Barnett, D. Shusman, K. Brown, F. Weidman-Dahl, and G. McDonnell. 1982. COSTAR: A comprehensive medical information system for ambulatory care. Pp. 8-18 in *Proceedings of the Sixth Symposium on Computer Applications in Medical Care*, ed. B. I. Blum. Washington, D.C.: IEEE Computer Society Press.

Benda, C. 1989. Are doctors computer-compatible? Are computers physician-friendly? *Minnesota Medicine* 3:146-150.

Blau, M. L. 1990. Emergency physicians gain malpractice discount. *Physicians News Digest* 6:2-3.

Bleich, H. L., and W. V. Slack. 1989. Clinical computing. *M.D. Computing* 6:133-135.

Bleich, H. L., C. Safran, and W. V. Slack. 1989. Departmental and laboratory computing in two hospitals. *M.D. Computing* 6:149-155.

Blum, B. I., ed. 1984. *Information Systems for Patient Care.* New York: Springer-Verlag.

Blum, B. I., ed. 1986. *Clinical Information Systems.* New York: Springer-Verlag.

Canfield, K., B. Bray, and S. Huff. 1990. Representation and database design for clinical information. Pp. 350-353 in *Proceedings of the Fourteenth Symposium on Computer Applications in Medical Care*, ed. R. A. Miller. Washington, D.C.: IEEE Computer Society Press.

Dayhoff, R. E., D. L. Maloney, and P. M. Kuzmak. 1990. Examination of architectures to allow integration of image data with hospital information systems. Pp. 694-698 in *Proceedings of the Fourteenth Symposium on Computer Applications in Medical Care*, ed. R. A. Miller. Washington, D.C.: IEEE Computer Society Press.

Friedman, C., G. Hripcsak, S. B. Johnson, J. J. Cimino, and P. D. Clayton. 1990. A generalized relational scheme for an integrated clinical patient database. Pp. 335-339 in *Proceedings of the Fourteenth Annual Symposium on Computer Applications in Medical Care,* ed. R. A. Miller. Washington, D.C.: IEEE Computer Society Press.

GAO (General Accounting Office). 1988. Use of Information Technology in Hospitals. Statement of Melroy D. Quasney, Associate Director, Information Management and Technology Division, before the Subcommittee on Education and Health, Joint Economic Committee. T-IMTEC-88-4. Washington, D.C. May 24.

GAO. 1990. Defense's Acquisition of the Composite Health Care System. Statement of Daniel C. White, Special Assistant to the Assistant Comptroller General, before the Subcommittee on Military Personnel and Compensation, Committee on Armed Services, U.S. House of Representatives. T-IMTEC-90-04. March 15.

Giebink, G. A., and L. L. Hurst. 1975. *Computer Projects in Health Care.* Ann Arbor, Mich.: Health Administration Press.

Greenes, R. A., and E. H. Shortliffe. 1990. Medical informatics: An emerging discipline and institutional priority. *Journal of the American Medical Association* 263:1114-1120.

Grossman, J. H., G. O. Barnett, and T. D. Koespell. 1973. An automated medical record system. *Journal of the American Medical Association* 224:1616-1621.

Hammond, W. E., and W. W. Stead. 1986. The evolution of a computerized medical information system. Pp. 147-156 in *Proceedings of the Tenth Symposium on Computer Applications in Medical Care,* ed. H. F. Orthner. New York: IEEE Computer Society Press.

Hammond, W. E., M. J. Straube, and W. W. Stead. 1990. The synchronization of distributed databases. Pp. 345-349 in *Proceedings of the Fourteenth Annual Symposium on Computer Applications in Medical Care,* ed. R. A. Miller. Washington, D.C.: IEEE Computer Society Press.

Harvard Community Health Plan. N.d. Automated Medical Record System (unpublished overview). Harvard Community Health Plan, Brookline, Mass.

Hopkins, R. J. 1990. The Exeter care card: A CPB-based global health care record for the United Kingdom's national health care service. *Journal of Medical Systems* 14:150-154.

Hripcsak, G., P. D. Clayton, T. A. Pryor, P. Haug, O. B. Wigertz, and J. Van der Lei. 1990. The Arden syntax for medical logic modules. Pp. 200-204 in *Proceedings of the Fourteenth Annual Symposium on Computer Applications in Medical Care,* ed. R. A. Miller. Washington, D.C.: IEEE Computer Society Press.

Humphreys, B. L., and D. A. B. Lindberg. 1989. Building the unified medical language system. Pp. 475-480 in *Proceedings of the Thirteenth Annual Symposium on Computer Applications in Medical Care,* ed. L. C. Kingsland. New York: IEEE Computer Society Press.

Kaufman, A., and J. Holbrook. 1990. *The Computer as Expert.* Springfield, Mass.: Mercy Hospital.

Kirby, J. D., M. P. Pickett, W. Boyarsky, and W. W. Stead. 1987. Distributed processing with a mainframe-based hospital information system: A generalized solution. *Proceedings of the Eleventh Annual Symposium on Computer Applications in Medical Care,* ed. W. W. Stead. Washington, D.C.: IEEE Computer Society Press.

Krakauer, H. 1990. The uniform clinical data set. Pp. 120-123 in *Effectiveness and Outcomes in Health Care,* ed. K. A. Heithoff and K. N. Lohr. Washington, D.C.: National Academy Press.

Ledley, R. S., and L. B. Lusted. 1960. The use of electronic computers in medical data processing. *IRE Transactions in Medical Electronics* 7:31-47.

Lindberg, D. A. B., and B. L. Humphreys. 1990. The UMLS knowledge sources: Tools for building better user interfaces. Pp. 121-125 in *Proceedings of the Fourteenth Annual Symposium on Computer Applications in Medical Care*, ed. R. A. Miller. Washington, D.C.: IEEE Computer Society Press.

Mandell, S. F. 1987. Resistance to computerization: An examination of the relationship between resistance and the cognitive style of the clinician. *Journal of Medical Systems* 4:311-318.

Margulies, D. M., R. Ribitzy, A. Elkowitz, and D. P. McCallie. 1989. Implementing an integrated hospital information system at Children's Hospital. Pp. 627-631 in *Proceedings of the Thirteenth Annual Symposium on Computer Applications in Medical Care*, ed. L. C. Kingsland. New York: IEEE Computer Society Press.

McDonald, C. J., L. Blevins, W. M. Tierney, and D. K. Martin. 1988. The Regenstrief medical records. *M.D. Computing* 5:34-47.

Miller, R. A., M. A. McNeil, S. M. Challinor, F. E. Masarie, and J. D. Myers. 1986. Status report. The INTERNIST-I: Quick medical reference project. *Western Journal of Medicine* 145:816-822.

National Research Council. 1991. *Computers at Risk: Safe Computing in the Information Age.* Washington, D.C.: National Academy Press.

Obermeier, K. 1989. *Natural Language Processing Technologies in Artificial Intelligence: The Science and Industry Perspective.* London: Ellis Horwood Limited.

Pryor, T. A., R. M. Gardner, P. D. Clayton, and H. R. Warner. 1983. The HELP system. *Journal of Medical Systems* 7:87-102.

Pryor, T. A., R. M. Gardner, P. D. Clayton, and H. R. Warner. 1984. The HELP system. Pp. 109-128 in *Information Systems for Patient Care*, ed. B. I. Blum. New York: Springer-Verlag.

Safran, C., D. Porter, J. Lightfoot, C. D. Rury, L. H. Underhill, H. L. Bleich, and W. V. Slack. 1989. ClinQuery: A system for online searching of data in a teaching hospital. *Annals of Internal Medicine* 111:751-756.

Scherrer, J. R., R. H. Baud, D. Hochstrasser, and R. Osman. 1990. An integrated hospital information system in Geneva. *M.D. Computing* 7:81-89.

Shortliffe, E. H. 1987. Computer programs to support clinical decision making. *Journal of the American Medical Association* 258:61-66.

Silva, J. S., A. J. Zawilski, and J. O'Brian. 1990. The physician workstation: An intelligent "front end" to a hospital information system. Pp. 764-767 in *Proceedings of the Fourteenth Symposium on Computer Applications in Medical Care*, ed. R. A. Miller. Washington, D.C.: IEEE Computer Society Press.

Slack, W. V. 1989. The soul of a new system: A modern parable. *M.D. Computing* 6:137-140.

Spencer, W. A., and C. Vallbona. 1965. Applications of computers in clinical practice. *Journal of the American Medical Association* 191:121-125.

Stead, W. W., and W. E. Hammond. 1987. Demand-oriented medical records: Toward a physician workstation. Pp. 275-280 in *Proceedings of the Eleventh Annual Symposium on Computer Applications in Medical Care*, ed. W. W. Stead. Washington, D.C.: IEEE Computer Society Press.

Stead, W. W., and W. E. Hammond. 1988. Computer-based medical records: The centerpiece of TMR. *M.D. Computing* 5:48-62.

Summerfield, A. B., and E. Empey. 1965. *Computer-based Information Systems for Medicine: A Survey and Brief Discussion of Current Projects.* Santa Monica, Calif.: Systems Development Corporation.

Walker, H. K. 1989. Grady Memorial's integrated database. *Computers in Healthcare* March:36-42.

Warner, H. R., C. M. Olmsted, and B. D. Rutherford. 1972. HELP: A program for medical decision-making. *Computers and Biomedical Research* 5:65.

Weed, L. L. 1968. Medical records that guide and teach. *New England Journal of Medicine* 278:593-600, 652-657.

Weed, L. L. (in press). *New Premises and New Tools for Medical Practice and Medical Education.* New York: Springer-Verlag.

Whiting-O'Keefe, Q. E., A. Whiting, and J. Henke. 1988. The STOR clinical information system. *M.D. Computing* 5:48-62.

Wiederhold, G. 1986. Views, objects and databases. *Computer* 19:37-44.

Wilton, R. W., and J. M. McCoy. 1989. Outpatient clinic information system based on distributed database technology. Pp. 372-376 in *Proceedings of the Thirteenth Symposium on Computer Applications in Medical Care*, ed. L. C. Kingsland. New York: IEEE Computer Society.

Young, D. W. 1987. What makes doctors use computers? Discussion Paper. Pp. 8-14 in *Use and Impact of Computers in Clinical Medicine*, ed. J. G. Anderson and S. J. Jay. New York: Springer-Verlag.

Zibrak, J. D., M. S. Roberts, L. Nelick-Cohen, and M. Peterson. 1990. Creating an environment conducive to physician participation in a hospital information system. Pp. 779-783 in *Proceedings of the Fourteenth Symposium on Computer Applications in Medical Care*, ed. R. A. Miller. Washington, D.C.: IEEE Computer Society Press.

APPENDIX:
THE COMPUTER-BASED PATIENT RECORD SYSTEM VENDOR SURVEY

The members of the Institute of Medicine study committee agreed that their deliberations would be enhanced by access to data on commercial clinical information systems and on the perspectives of those who develop and market them. The committee's Technology Subcommittee therefore conducted an informal survey to solicit basic information from vendors active in the computer-based patient record system market. Twelve vendors associated with clinical information systems (including three hardware manufacturers) responded. This appendix briefly summarizes findings and conclusions derived by the subcommittee from the responses to the survey.

General Observations

The range of responses, both to the survey as a whole and to the individual items within it, indicated substantial differences among members of the software development industry about the operational definition of the computer-based patient record and the data that should be captured in it. Vendor responses suggested that the industry viewed direct data entry as desirable, but they also reflected industry pessimism about whether physicians and nurses could be convinced to actually enter data (although three vendors stated that they had implemented systems in which direct data entry by practitioners was occurring). Other impediments to the immediate implementation of CPRs today, as opposed to in the future, included the cost of the system, general resistance to change within the health care industry, the need for data sharing among many different kinds of systems (including departmental systems), and the lack of a good decision support system.

Vendors showed more agreement in their view of the forces that could propel the medical record environment into the computer age. Most cited the increasingly broad range of medical record users, which mandates a patient record with expanded access. Strong consensus emerged regarding the CPR as a tool with the potential to benefit every aspect of the health care environment. Vendors also voiced some skepticism, however, that the CPR could receive the broad-based, organization-wide support required for its implementation and use in a hospital.

According to the vendor responses, technologies commonly believed to be 5 to 10 years distant are, in fact, already being employed in workable CPR systems. Three vendors claimed that they had implemented a full-scale electronic medical record in a hospital environment: one in a facility of unspecified size, the second in a hospital of 176 beds, and the third in a large, urban teaching hospital of more than 900 beds. Two of these vendors offered decision support systems, one of which was described as a powerful report-writing system and the other as an actual interactive decision support system. The survey responses also indicated that direct data entry by patient care practitioners was feasible, resistance to change notwithstanding, provided the CPR system was user friendly and was perceived as improving quality and reducing costs for the hospital, clinic, or practice. Taken together, the survey responses appeared to suggest that the environment is right for the implementation of CPRs in hospitals—that is, if enough of the system's beneficiaries can be convinced that such a comprehensive system justifies the difficulties of implementation.

Survey Findings

FINDING 1. Close reading of the responses generates some skepticism about whether all of the named products meet the requirements of a comprehensive CPR system. This may be the case in part because too few of the necessary patient record components have been automated.

FINDING 2. The majority of the systems noted in the survey operate in multiprocessor environments, a configuration that arises in response to a hospital's demands for flexible implementation and system expandability. This trend can be expected to continue. All but one of the systems are designed to run on the hardware of a particular vendor; the exception is a system adaptable to any hardware that uses UNIX. For the most part, the systems described in the survey do not employ the most advanced terminal technologies, even though these technologies are no longer new on the market. The one exception to this generalization—the vendor whose product is adaptable to many different types of computer hardware—supports both windowing and point-and-click technologies.

FINDING 3. System costs, including installation, are likely to be in the range of $2 million to $6 million for a medium-sized hospital. Annual maintenance costs for each system could be substantial—approximately 10 percent of the purchase or lease price.

FINDING 4. With the exception of a single software vendor, the industry is moving slowing in solving one crucial problem: ease of data entry. Although such devices as the mouse and the light pen are commonly used in other industries, and even in home computing, they are rarely found in health care computing. The only vendor that offers evidence of having solved the problem of convincing physicians and nurses to use the system is the same vendor that has exploited these technologies most fully. The same conclusion may be drawn with regard to flexible output devices: the vendor that offers the most flexible data-entry methods also supports the most varied output, including terminal windowing, and has the most flexible hardware requirements.

FINDING 5. The survey responses are informative regarding vendor *attitudes* toward the state of the art in CPR systems, but they may not be helpful in defining the *actual* state of the art. The committee found it surprising that the software vendors who responded to the survey should so heavily emphasize hardware improvements as the necessary step in advancing to comprehensive CPRs and CPR systems.

FINDING 6. The last set of findings was based on a group of open-ended questions to which only a few vendors responded. In general, they seem reluctant to lay out in detail imaginative ideas regarding the impact of computerized systems on the industry their systems are intended to serve, namely, the health care industry. Thus, the committee found it disturbing that the vendors appeared pessimistic, perhaps unintentionally, about surmounting the difficulties involved in implementing the CPR—especially given the success that some have had in overcoming certain technological and behavioral problems associated with CPR implementation.

4

The Road to CPR Implementation

Technological change is a complex process that is influenced by a multitude of factors, including the attributes of a technology, the users of the technology, and the environment in which the technology is used. Successful implementation of computer-based patient record systems depends on "more than the transmission of technical details and the availability of systems" (Anderson and Jay, 1987:4). It requires an understanding of the factors that influence the development and adoption of computer technologies in health care.

This chapter first identifies the factors that could enhance or impede CPR development and use. It then presents the committee's plan for addressing these factors. The plan includes a discussion of the various organizations that have a role to play in CPR development and diffusion, the types of activities that would facilitate patient record development, how such activities might be implemented, and when such activities should take place. Chapter 5 presents the committee's formal recommendations for achieving the primary goals of the plan.

DEVELOPMENT AND DIFFUSION FACTORS

The process of technological change involves two general stages: development and diffusion. Development is the production of new capabilities or the alteration of characteristics of existing technologies; diffusion is the application of a new technology in the provision of services. These two stages do not necessarily occur in chronological sequence. User application can reveal that a technology needs further development. Alternatively, diffusion sometimes parallels the development of a new technology (NAS, 1979). Moreover, as discussed below, the factors affecting development and diffusion are interrelated: development is unlikely to occur if the conditions for diffusion are unfavorable.

Barriers to Development

Patient Record Definition

A basic impediment to the development of CPRs and CPR systems has been the lack of a clear definition of what a CPR could and should be. An intellectual understanding of what a CPR needs to do, the range of individuals for whom it needs to function, and the expectations and performance demands of its users is an essential prerequisite to successful design of a CPR system (Teach and Shortliffe, 1981). Many computer-based information management systems are currently in place and generate and use patient data for various purposes (e.g., billing, laboratory, radiology); what is lacking is a unified concept of what constitutes a computer-based patient record system.

A fully articulated definition of a CPR and CPR system should describe attributes of the record and system (i.e., content, format, and function) as a guide for system developers and users.[1] It should not, however, prescribe how those attributes are to be achieved. Resolution of that question is best left to CPR system developers and vendors.

Chapter 2 identifies basic CPR system requirements, but system designers require more detailed specification in certain areas. Among these are the level of performance (e.g., speed and convenience) the system must provide to achieve health care provider acceptance; the kinds of new system functions needed to justify a change in current routines of record use and the costs of implementation; the frequency with which multiple users would view the record simultaneously; the level of system security, confidentiality, and reliability required; and the level of institutional, regional, national, or international interconnectivity demanded of the system.

In particular, patient record system developers require specific information about system functionality and performance to design systems that meet user needs. Understanding the diverse set of CPR user needs requires that representatives of all users be involved in a process of setting priorities for system functionality and performance.

---

[1]As discussed in Chapter 1, the committee's definition of a CPR is an electronic patient record that resides in a system specifically designed to support users through the availability of complete, accurate patient data, alerts, reminders, clinical decision support systems, links to medical knowledge, and other aids.

Content and Format Standards

As discussed in Chapter 3, CPR development has been, and continues to be, impeded by the lack of standards for the content and format of CPR data (McDonald and Hammond, 1989; Bradbury, 1990; Gabrieli and Murphy, 1990; Lindberg and Humphreys, 1990; Masys, 1990). To exploit the potential benefits of linking CPRs across specialties and institutions, developers must ensure the following. (1) The content of CPRs must be defined; that is, each CPR should contain a uniform core set of data elements. (2) Data elements must be named consistently; that is, some form of vocabulary control must be in place. (3) Format standards for data exchange must be developed and used.

Defining a core set of data elements requires participation by representatives of all patient record user groups. (Exclusion of any group could diminish the efficiency to be gained from implementing CPR systems if, as a result, key data elements are excluded from the core data set.) However, the uniform core data set should not be so large that it requires health care professionals to collect information that does not derive directly from routine service provision. Moreover, because providers are likely to require data elements in addition to those in the uniform core data set, CPR systems should be flexible and not be limited to core data elements.

Vocabulary control efforts have already led to substantial progress in developing standardized vocabularies. The use of existing controlled vocabularies in combination could cover the basic name of each patient problem and of each procedure performed by a practitioner (Lindberg and Humphreys, 1990). Inadequate support for the timely update of clinical vocabularies, however, remains an obstacle to developing better vocabulary control for the CPR. Another obstacle is user resistance: users generally have not considered the benefits of a reasonably specific, controlled vocabulary as warranting a switch to a new system—especially if that system entails higher costs for record creation and maintenance (Lindberg and Humphreys, 1990).

Existing format standards focus on particular portions of the record; no single format standard exists that could be used for the entire CPR. Nor is there at present a means for establishing one standard for use by the entire health care industry. In short, format standards for data exchange need further development and a means of achieving credibility. To date, such efforts have been carried out primarily by volunteer organizations. Greater support (i.e., funding and recognition) of these efforts would help to accelerate standards development.

Costs and Risks

Venture capital is unlikely to be forthcoming for large-scale technological systems that require sizable investments before yielding a return in a highly uncertain market (NAS, 1979). Consequently, development of a technology may require subsidization of development costs or creation of a more certain market, or both (NAS, 1979). Both of these factors apply to CPR systems: they require significant investment for development, and a high degree of uncertainty exists regarding the willingness of health care providers to purchase the systems.

As discussed in Chapter 3, the committee found no comprehensive CPR systems in existence in 1990. Furthermore, no cost data are available on the monetary investment that might be required to implement such a system; evaluations of cost data related to computer applications tend to have focused on medical information systems (MISs) rather than on CPR systems. MIS development costs and time estimates, however, do convey a sense of the magnitude of CPR development costs and time. A survey of automated ambulatory care systems found that development costs ranged from $100,000 to $10 million and that development time ranged from 1 to 7 years (Henley and Wiederhold, 1975). Congress's Office of Technology Assessment (OTA) has estimated the development cost for a commercial inpatient MIS to be $25 million and the time to develop such a system to be 10 years (OTA, 1977). Costs related to the acquisition of a technology are discussed later in this chapter.

A General Accounting Office (GAO) study on the use of information technology in hospitals found that commercial hospital information systems currently in use were not as comprehensive as those planned by the Department of Defense and the Department of Veterans Affairs (GAO, 1988). The GAO cited two factors that could account for the less extensive development of commercial information systems—which may itself reflect an uncertain market. The first is the potentially small market for such systems.[2] The second is the low level of spending for automation in the hospital industry. The causes of this low level are uncertain, but GAO offers several possibilities: the historical lack of incentives for hospitals to minimize costs (a situation that has changed since the implementation of the prospective payment system by Medicare); the difficulties hospitals face in trying to raise initial funds for information systems; the cost savings in early systems were attributed to reductions in the work of clerical rather than clinical staff; the difficulties involved in achieving or quantifying savings (time savings in particular are likely to be fragmented); and resistance by medical personnel to the introduction of information management technology (GAO, 1987).

---

[2]Some experts believe hospitals must have 200 or more operating beds to make optimal use of hospital information systems. According to the GAO report (1988), nearly 70 percent of community hospitals have fewer than 200 operating beds.

The CPR market may also be uncertain because computer applications are generally not well understood by health care practitioners (Anderson and Jay, 1987). This lack of understanding limits the demand for such products and, as a result, reduces commercial interest in developing new products. Few sources exist to help practitioners learn what a computer technology can do for them, and there is little likelihood such help will be forthcoming in the near future, given the costs associated with producing such resources.

Barriers to Diffusion

Technological diffusion has been analyzed in greater depth than technological development. Rogers (1987) presents five characteristics of a technology that influence its adoption:

• relative advantage over existing technologies (the degree to which an innovation is perceived as better than the practice it supersedes);
• compatibility (the degree to which an innovation is perceived to be consistent with values, experiences, and needs of potential adopters, as well as with the structure of adopting organizations);
• complexity (the degree to which an innovation is perceived as difficult to understand and use);
• feasibility[3] (the degree to which one can experiment with an innovation on a limited basis); and
• observability (the degree to which the results of an innovation are observable to others).

Other factors also affect CPR adoption and use, including the environment of the health care system; leadership; user behavior, education, and training; costs; social and legal issues; and network needs. Major concerns in these areas are briefly noted below.

Environment of the Health Care System

The U.S. health care system has been characterized as comprising "thousands of relatively autonomous units, centering on large hospitals, which are themselves made up of relatively autonomous divisions and departments" (Lindberg, 1979:215). Maintaining CPRs, however, "imposes requirements for greater coordination among separate ancillary services, particularly with regard to terminology" (McDonald and Tierney, 1988:3438).

---

[3]Rogers (1987) uses the term *trialability* to reflect the degree to which an innovation can be experimented with on a limited basis.

By extension, the use of patient records that are linkable requires coordination among the institutions that are likely to contribute to or use such records. Thus, autonomy within and among provider institutions must be addressed when planning and implementing CPR systems.

Disaggregation of care (i.e., the delivery of medical care by many small providers who operate independently of and in competition with one another) has significant implications for the adoption of a coordinative, systemwide technology. Such technology is often subject to nonadditive benefits—that is, the benefits of collaboration among multiple providers outweigh the benefits of individual adoption. As a result, providers have fewer incentives to acquire such technology (NAS, 1979).

The reimbursement policies that are applied to providers influence their willingness and ability to acquire CPR technology. For instance, under cost-based reimbursement schemes, providers have more incentive to acquire technologies that are reimbursable than technologies that are not reimbursable. In contrast, prospective payment systems create incentives for institutions to reduce costs—and thus to acquire potentially cost-reducing technologies such as CPR systems. Under current reimbursement policies, any potential acquisition of new technology must contribute to the improvement of a provider's financial status or at least be budget neutral. It should also substantially improve patient care processes, for example, by providing clinical decision support or by giving complete record access to authorized personnel.

Leadership

Given the fragmented environment of the U.S. health care system, it is not surprising that at present no one organization or agency is leading the effort to establish the necessary infrastructure for national implementation of CPRs and CPR systems. National and regional organizations may be knowledgeable about the issues, but they are not consistently soliciting information from or educating their members about CPRs. Thus, despite the many aspects of CPRs that are in need of coordination, no organization has the operational responsibility and funds to establish programs and projects to set the direction for the health care industry. Overcoming this problem could be the key requirement for progress, and the committee devoted considerable attention to discussing and formulating its primary recommendation in this area (see Chapter 5).

User Behavior, Education, and Training

Users are more likely to accept a technology if several conditions are met: they have a stake in the system; they can use it at minimum cost; the technology produces information leading to improved clinical services; that information is almost immediately available; and the technology increases their status (Young, 1987). Computing applications that do not significantly change the routines associated with the practice of medicine are also more likely to be accepted by users (Kaplan, 1987).

An individual's propensity to use a technology has been attributed to specialization, fear of malpractice suits, industry promotion, a specific form of medical practice, and payment methods (Banta, 1987). An encounter with a peer who is already using a technology can also influence an individual's use (Anderson et al., 1987).

Young (1987:9) suggests that problems with the acceptance of clinical computing systems relate to the way a physician organizes his or her thought processes and interacts with written aids.

> [U]se of the medical records is not properly appreciated. The written record is not just a repository of information; it often forms part of the doctor's thought process, so that the style of writing, the position on the paper of particular items, abbreviations, the sequence of information, use of margins, may all have an important significance for the individual practitioner—a significance which goes beyond the actual facts recorded, and which is impossible to capture in an orderly typed record or video display unit. It is the loss of these individual aspects of the medical record which causes most problems. The advantages of structured, typewritten reports commonly do not outweigh the loss of the extra information which is conveyed to the individual practitioner by the above features.

Some individuals in the health care community are skeptical that computer systems can be designed to meet user performance and functional requirements. They may also doubt that a CPR system will improve an institution's ability to manage its information. Previous negative experiences with computer systems or inaccurate data generated by a system may cause some providers to actively resist the acquisition and implementation of CPRs. Whether or not an individual clinician is skeptical about a CPR system, using it will require behavioral changes. Thus, as noted earlier, some natural resistance to the CPR is to be expected.

Individual institutions will need educational programs to support these changes. Educational curricula for health care professionals must also be modified to reflect the role of the CPR in the provision of health care services. Who will develop, implement, and pay for such materials (e.g., vendors or professional groups) is an area of considerable uncertainty.

CPR implementation requires experts who can support CPR users, but at present only a relatively small number of individuals have the necessary expertise in medical informatics (Clepper, 1991). More people must be encouraged to enter this field and a variety of educational and training programs tailored to different types of health care professionals must be developed. The committee considered the educational barrier to CPR development sufficiently important to formulate a specific recommendation to address it, as discussed in Chapter 5.

In addition to education, practitioners need incentives to use CPRs to enter data and maintain patient records. Perhaps the greatest motivation for practitioners to use CPRs would be to produce evidence that CPRs can help to improve the quality of patient care and reduce the administrative burdens they currently face. As discussed in Chapter 3, at least one institution has experimented with a fee-for-data arrangement for physicians who input their own discharge summaries into an automated system. Other arrangements to encourage the use of CPRs are also feasible. For example, third-party payers could provide incentives for health care providers (including physicians) to submit claims electronically or in a computer-compatible format (e.g., diskette). Alternatively, third-party payers may reject reimbursement claims that do not contain standard data. A regulatory approach is another possibility for use in place of or in addition to an incentive structure. However, the potential side effects and costs of both incentives and constrictive regulations must be understood and carefully weighed.

Costs

A major factor influencing a firm's adoption of a technology is the size of the investment required relative to the size of the firm. Acquisition costs for CPR systems are likely to be substantial but are difficult to estimate.[4] This difficulty arises because the purchase or lease price of a system does not reflect the total implementation cost; it excludes the cost of training and potential losses of productivity during transition to the system. Studies that have attempted to estimate total costs have tended to focus on MISs rather than CPR systems. Further, purchase or lease prices for CPR systems vary significantly, depending on the scope of functions a system offers, the size of an institution, and an institution's previous level of automation.

One cost analysis of the implementation and operation of an automated ambulatory care medical record system found that the cost per patient encounter of a computer-based system was 26 percent greater than the direct costs associated with operation of a manual system. However, the manual system failed to access 18 percent of the records requested within the de-

---

[4]A confidential survey of CPR vendors conducted by the Technology Subcommittee of this IOM study committee revealed that purchase or lease costs for a CPR system range from $2 million to $6 million for a medium-sized hospital (see the appendix to Chapter 3).

mand time, whereas the automated system provided access to 100 percent of the records requested. Quantification of the access benefit reduced the difference in costs between the two systems (Koster et al., 1987).

This cost analysis illustrates another major difficulty faced by health care provider institutions deciding on acquisition of a CPR system. Decisions about whether to acquire technology are based in part on information about the benefits of the technology; once again, data on CPR system benefits are sparse. Few recent studies have analyzed actual costs and benefits. The studies that have been conducted address MISs rather than CPR systems; they also focus on projected rather than actual experience or include only those benefits that can be measured in terms of dollars and exclude such benefits as improved quality of care or reduced waiting time for patients.

The costs of acquiring and operating CPRs and CPR systems will be borne primarily by practitioners and health care provider institutions. Yet the benefits of these systems will accrue to patients, practitioners, health care provider institutions, third-party payers, researchers, policymakers, and the public. These cumulative benefits of CPR systems should exceed the benefits individual practitioners and health care providers might be expected to gain. As such, CPR systems in certain respects represent a public good.

Given today's strict budget constraints, health care provider institutions (including physicians' offices) must choose among alternative technologies when allocating resources. Compared with a CPR system, other technologies could offer greater monetary benefits to an individual institution, albeit lower combined or social (public good) benefits. When this situation prevails, provider institutions have fewer incentives to invest in CPRs and CPR systems.

Nonclinical data users (e.g., third-party payers and researchers) could also incur costs from CPR implementation. They may need to modify existing systems or acquire new ones to be compatible with CPR standards; they may also need to revise procedures for handling computer-based data and develop training programs for personnel.

The cost of CPR technology, like the cost of computer technology in general, may well decrease over time. Moreover, CPRs may reduce the costs of care enough to offset the expense of acquiring and operating CPR systems, although this remains to be proved. The committee was quite concerned about the immediate barriers to CPR implementation raised by potentially substantial costs for full acquisition, installation, and operation of CPR systems across the nation; it was also concerned about the distribution of these costs. Consequently, it formulated a specific recommendation to address these matters, which is presented in Chapter 5.

Legal and Social Issues

The legal and social issues involved in implementing CPRs and CPR systems are formidable. State licensure requirements for hospital medical records are obsolete, ambiguous, and nonuniform (Waller, in this volume). The wide variation among states in hospital licensure requirements for medical records makes it difficult to develop CPR systems that comply with licensure laws in all 50 states; this factor in turn hinders the development of CPR formats that can be used nationally. Failure by a vendor to establish a CPR system's compliance with one or more state licensure requirements may adversely affect the system's marketability. The differences across states could be so great as to make national implementation impossible.

Hospital licensure laws and regulations in some states still assume a paper patient record, which makes the legal status of CPR systems unclear. Other state laws and regulations appear to permit use of some forms of automation but not others, or the use of automation for some, but not all, patient record functions. It is not clear whether regulations requiring that records be kept in ink or be typewritten permit the creation of records electronically or the use of lasers. Further, the regulations in many states require that medical records be signed but are silent on whether a computer key or code can be substituted for a signature.

Issues of record ownership, responsibility, and control must also be addressed. The physical records are the property of the provider institution at which they were created. In addition, provider institutions currently are responsible for ensuring the accuracy and completeness of record contents (Amatayakul and Wogan, 1989). As data are transmitted and shared among institutions, all with the ability to add and update information from a variety of settings, the principles of ownership become blurred. It is not clear who would maintain records for routine use and maintain the structure of the record to accommodate new terminology and data elements for new diseases, treatments, tests, and approaches to health care. The locus of control of access to patient data is another unanswered question. Current laws concerning disclosure of and access to patient record information vary from state to state, further complicating the transfer of patient information across state lines.

Perhaps the impediment to CPRs that is of greatest concern is the issue of privacy. The computerization of most types of record keeping, as well as the recent well-publicized cases of inappropriate access by computer hackers, has increased concerns about the misuse of personal information (Westin, 1976; Privacy Protection Study Commission, 1977; Peck, 1984; Agranoff, 1989). A system in which patient data, including sensitive information (e.g., human immunodeficiency virus test results, data on psychiatric treatment), can be accessed more easily may be strongly resisted in some quarters.[5]

There are several aspects to concerns about confidentiality of information and patient privacy. Ultimate responsibility for protecting the privacy of patient data that are shared among multiple users has not been defined; in addition, generally accepted standards for the protection of computer-based data do not exist (Agranoff, 1989; NRC, 1991). The consequences for breaches of confidentiality vary by state and in some cases need to be stronger than they are at present (Waller, in this volume). The National Conference of Commissioners on Uniform State Laws drafted the Uniform Health-Care Information Act to address issues of patient privacy, patient access, disclosure of patient information to third parties, and transfer of such information across state lines (National Conference of Commissioners on Uniform State Laws, 1986). As of this writing, however, only one state had adopted this act (Waller, in this volume).

Concerns about patient privacy affect more than the security features of CPR systems and legal remedies. A consistent personal identification number (PIN) in all patient records would facilitate record linkage across time and provider institutions (National Center for Health Statistics, 1990; Washington Business Group on Health, 1989). Nevertheless, despite its operational attractiveness to researchers and other patient record users, the PIN raises concerns about the increased potential to invade patient privacy (Washington Business Group on Health, 1989).

Currently, the Food and Drug Administration (FDA) device regulations and authorities do not apply to computer products intended only for use

---

[5]Westin's 1976 study of the impact on citizen rights of computers in the health care field found that "most cases of *actual harm* involving individuals were still arising from manual records" and concluded that the main problem with the use of computer-based patient records involved "*potential harm*—the creation of health data systems that many health professionals, citizen groups, and individuals directly affected by such systems consider to be *threats* to basic rights" (Westin, 1976:xvi, emphasis in original). As noted by Lindberg (1970), however, the public and its elected legislators must have their anxieties allayed about potential misuses of data.

Some observers have suggested that computer-based patient record systems will offer greater confidentiality for patient information because they can limit the information that various users can see. For example, administrative or financial personnel could be prevented from seeing sensitive diagnostic or treatment data. Further, CPR systems could provide an audit trail listing those personnel who accessed a particular record (Hard, 1990).

As discussed in Chapter 3, however, existing security technology frequently has been not applied to current CPR systems. Moreover, a recent National Research Council (NRC) study on computer system security concerns concluded that several trends reflected a growing potential for system abuse. Among these trends are the proliferation of networking and embedded systems, the widespread use of databases containing personal information, and the widespread ability to use and abuse computers (NRC, 1991).

in such traditional library functions as storage, retrieval, and dissemination of medical information (Food and Drug Administration, 1989). As of this writing, however, the FDA's policy on the regulation of computer products had not been finalized; this situation creates uncertainty for vendors about potential regulation and its effects on system development costs and time.

Liability for system defects is also a concern of vendors, particularly given the still-developing field of medical computer liability (Brannigan and Dayhoff, 1986; Willick, 1986; Metzger, 1988; Denis and Poullet, 1990). It has been asserted that a strict liability is likely to be applied to system vendors in cases in which the computer produces output on which a physician relies without further checking, for example, patient record systems (Brannigan and Dayhoff, 1986; Bronzino et al., 1990).

Liability for defects in clinical decision support systems is less clearly defined. System developers (i.e., health care specialists and computer programmers), manufacturers, purchasers, and users are all involved in bringing a computer system to the patient. In cases in which harm is caused, liability could be assigned if negligence (i.e., lack of due care) can be proved and if the patient can prove that the negligent party owed a duty of care to the patient. (Physicians already have an established duty of care to patients.) Practitioners are expected to use such systems to supplement the medical library or to act in place of a consultant; they can ignore information provided by such systems and are expected to evaluate its accuracy. Thus, liability for negligence in the use of clinical decision support systems could apply to practitioners.[6]

The nature and obduracy of the legal barriers to CPR implementation must be understood, underscored, and addressed. For that reason, Appendix B discusses legal aspects of computer-based patient records and record systems. Among the more critical legal aspects addressed there are regulatory and accreditation issues, evidentiary issues, patient privacy and record access concerns, record ownership questions, legal risks attached to specific CPR systems, and computer contracting issues. The committee regarded these issues as significant obstacles and formulated a specific recommendation to address legal barriers (see Chapter 5).

Network Needs

To transmit and link records presumes the existence of an infrastructure, that is, a network and standards for data communication on the network.

---

[6]There has also been some discussion about the potential for practitioners to be found negligent if they do not use clinical decision support systems once the systems become widely available in the future (Willick, 1986; Metzger, 1988).

Both communications technology and a management structure to coordinate participants are necessary elements of a network. Currently, the necessary coordinative mechanisms and the resources to establish and operate a health care computer network are not available. Those in the health care field must, as a result, look to other established networks for data transmission.

Internet is a loosely organized confederation of federal, regional, and local networks that are used by researchers and educators for electronic mail, software and data file transfer, graphics and image file transfer, remote computer access to supercomputers and other specialized research instruments, and remote access to computerized databases.[7] An estimated 1 million researchers are active users of the academic networks that are connected to Internet. It does not, however, provide users with uniformity in the type and quality of service; furthermore, despite its size, Internet does not yet reach the entire research and education community (Gould, 1990a).

Federal sponsors and academic participants envision continued evolution of Internet until it becomes a user-friendly, unified high-speed research network with nationwide coverage. The Federal Networking Council[8] plans to transform Internet into a full-fledged National Research and Education Network (NREN) in three phases. The final phase calls for an operational national network with gigabit-capacity trunks and for transition of the network from government to commercial operation (Gould, 1990b).

The NREN is being built to support "communication and resource sharing among institutions and individuals engaged in unclassified research and scholarly pursuit" (Gould, 1990b:1). As such, it is a model for the kind of infrastructure needed to transmit patient record data routinely. Given the

---

[7]In 1969 the Defense Advanced Research Projects Agency (DARPA) established an experimental network to demonstrate the potential of computer networking based on packet-switching technology, which allows many users to share a common communications channel. During the 1970s, DARPA sponsored several additional networks and supported the development of a set of rules and procedures (called the Internet protocols) for addressing and routing messages across separate networks. In the 1980s, DARPA sought to separate the operational traffic and administrative burden of military research and development (MILNET) from that of general academic research needs (Internet). Since 1985, the National Science Foundation has been responsible for coordinating the development of Internet. Funding for operations comes from five federal agencies involved in operating research networks and from universities, states, and private companies that operate and participate in local and regional networks (Gould, 1990a).

[8]The Federal Networking Council includes representatives from DARPA, the Departments of Energy and Health and Human Services, the National Aeronautics and Space Administration, and the National Science Foundation (Gould, 1990a).

[9]Senate Bill S. 1067 (High-Performance Computing Act of 1990) authorized the expenditure of $95 million over three years by the National Science Foundation for research, development, and support of the National Research and Education Network (National Science Foundation, 1990).

magnitude of the resources required to establish a national network,[9] the committee recognized the utility of using the NREN to accommodate the data transmission needs of health care beyond simply research and education. The committee viewed planning for health care's high-speed network needs to be a key factor in CPR diffusion and proposes a specific approach for future efforts later in this chapter.

ELEMENTS OF AN IMPLEMENTATION STRATEGY

The remainder of this chapter outlines the elements of a strategy to foster nationwide implementation of CPRs and CPR systems within a decade. The discussion focuses first on change agents and stakeholders, moving on to resources and finally organizational structures. Specific committee recommendations directed toward particular aspects of this strategy are developed more fully in Chapter 5.

Change Agents and Stakeholders

The committee distinguished between potential change agents and stakeholders in the process of developing and implementing CPR systems. Change agents are individuals or organizations who have, first, a mandate related to or significant interest in CPR implementation and, second, the resources or means for effecting a change (e.g., leadership position, regulation, funding). Change agents are in a position to initiate and facilitate the change process.

Stakeholders are individuals or organizations who are affected positively or negatively (or both) by the change and who thus may support or oppose it accordingly. Potential impacts faced by stakeholders include, for example, financial gain or loss, a threat to professional autonomy, and an increased risk of loss of privacy. Although stakeholders may not initiate a change process or have the potential to advance a desired change, they may have the ability to thwart it.

Table 4-1 identifies the main organizations and groups of individuals who are potential change agents or stakeholders with respect to developing and implementing CPR systems. They are grouped by sector—public or private—and are further designated according to the scope of their primary influence (i.e., national, regional, local, or individual).

To engage the support of change agents in the change process, it is necessary to understand their interest level and available resources. To manage the change process, it is necessary to identify the potential impact of a change on stakeholders. The interests and resources of major CPR change agents and the potential impact on CPR stakeholders of the changes they might effect are discussed below.

TABLE 4-1   Change Agents and Stakeholders Important to the
Implementation of Computer-based Patient Record Systems

Organization	Change Agent/Scope of Influence	Stakeholder
Public Sector		
Agency for Health Care Policy and Research	Yes/national	Yes
Centers for Disease Control	No	Yes
Congress	Yes/national	Yes
Department of Defense	Yes/national	Yes
Department of Veterans Affairs	Yes/national	Yes
Food and Drug Administration	No	Yes
Health Resources and Services Administration	Yes/national	Yes
Health Care Financing Administration	Yes/national	Yes
National Institutes of Health	No	Yes
National Library of Medicine[a]	Yes/national	No
State health agencies	Yes/regional	Yes
State legislatures	Yes/regional	Yes
Private Sector		
Computer standards organizations	Yes/national	No
Computer-based patient record vendors	Yes/national	Yes
Health care professionals	Yes/individual	Yes
Joint Commission for Accreditation of Healthcare Organizations	Yes/national	No
Patients	No	Yes
Patient groups	Yes/local to national	Yes
Professional associations	Yes/national	Yes
Professional schools	Yes/regional to national	Yes
Provider institutions	Yes/local	Yes
Researchers	No	Yes
Third-party payers	Yes/local to national	Yes
Universities	Yes/regional to national	Yes

[a]A specific agency of the National Institutes of Health.

Health Care Professionals and Professional Associations

Health care professionals bear a dual burden: they must learn to use a new technology, and they must change their behavior. Some professionals may view the CPR as a threat to their professional roles and resist implementation of CPR systems through attempts at circumvention or even system sabotage (Dowling, 1987). Alternatively, professionals can support development and implementation by participating in planning and by influencing their peers.

Professional associations for physicians, nurses, dentists, social workers, physical therapists, and similar kinds of health care practitioners are all vehicles by which to provide ongoing education to their members about the benefits and liabilities of CPRs. Associations such as the American College of Physicians, American College of Surgeons, American Dental Association, American Hospital Association, American Medical Association, American Medical Record Association, American Nurses Association, and Group Health Association of America are among the societies that could implement formal CPR education and awareness programs as part of their membership mailings and annual meetings. Many already have active committees to deal with medical informatics issues.

These and similar associations are likely to voice the concerns of their members, but they are also in a position to influence their members. Depending on how they weigh the advantages and disadvantages of CPR activities, they can lobby for or against them. To the extent that professional organizations see more benefits than liabilities in CPR implementation, they can be valuable participants in future consensus-building activities.

Patients and Representatives of Patients

As discussed earlier, the question of ensuring privacy and confidentiality has been identified as one of the crucial hurdles to effective CPR implementation. Given patient concerns about privacy and the potential for CPR systems to increase information flow within and outside of health care provider settings, patients may distrust CPR systems. Furthermore, patients are no more likely than health care professionals to use or understand computers, let alone computer-based record systems.

Survey data suggest that Americans view the nation's health care system as poorly organized and inefficient; most believe that rising health care costs can be reduced without cutting the quality of care (Blendon, 1988). As noted elsewhere in this report, CPRs and CPR systems offer many advantages (compared with current paper records) for overcoming some of these inefficiencies and improving health care quality. Hence, patients may have some basis for supporting the implementation of CPR systems.

Any influence of individual patients on CPR efforts is likely to be indirect at best. Patients might, for example, select providers on the basis of the provider's use of a CPR system. Greater influence can be exerted by the various voluntary membership organizations that represent the concerns of particular patient groups (e.g., the American Diabetes Association) or those of specific population groups (e.g., the American Association of Retired Persons). These organizations have the capacity to acquire a broad understanding of the strengths and limitations of CPRs and CPR systems and to offer substantial support or opposition to CPR activities.

Provider Institutions

Health care provider institutions are likely to be interested in CPR systems in response to concerns about quality and costs and to internal and external demands for information. By purchasing a CPR system, provider institutions can influence CPR development and implementation in three ways. First, such action signals the market that demand for CPR systems exists. Second, it directly affects the staff who must use the system. Third, it can help to create an understanding on the part of both providers and patients that such systems are the emerging standard of practice.

Third-party Payers

Third-party payers include both insurers and employers. For insurers, CPR systems offer an opportunity to streamline operations. To realize the gains in efficiency and productivity offered by CPR systems, however, insurers may have to incur short-term costs to make their systems compatible with CPR formats. Long-term improvements in efficiency may also be realized; for instance, redundant data entry can be eliminated through electronic claims submission and payment.

Insurers have a major stake in improving the knowledge base for quality and cost management (e.g., clinical practice guidelines and utilization management), as well as for coverage and reimbursement decisions (e.g., technology assessment and outcomes research). As change agents, insurers could offer incentives—for example, faster payment of claims when they are submitted in electronic form. Alternatively, because third-party payers should value improved data, they could increase reimbursement rates to reflect the costs of implementing and operating CPR systems.

Employers are likely to be interested in CPRs as a means of improving the quality and reducing the costs of care received by their employees and related beneficiaries. Groups such as the U.S. Chamber of Commerce, the Washington Business Group on Health, and regional health care business coalitions have devoted considerable resources to finding ways to manage the utilization and cost of health care services, which are ultimately reflected in the health care insurance premiums employers pay. The potential for CPRs to improve information management at the micro (patient) and macro (population) levels is likely to be of interest to employers. Health care business coalitions, chambers of commerce, and major employers could all contribute to CPR development and implementation efforts by financially supporting research and pilot demonstrations and by developing relationships with insurers and health care provider institutions that use or support CPR systems.

Federal Government

EXECUTIVE AGENCIES   Federal agencies have varying degrees of interest in and authority to influence CPR development and implementation. Certain agencies can provide substantial funding for research and development; others may be able to finance the acquisition of CPR technology. Federal agencies can support standards development through funding or regulatory mandate. For instance, they can direct major federal providers of health care to use CPR equipment that meets certain standards, or they can require the use of CPR technology for hospital accreditation or Medicare participation. The remainder of this section outlines the change agent and stakeholder roles of selected federal departments and agencies.

Within the Department of Health and Human Services (DHHS), the Public Health Service agencies[10] would benefit greatly from efficient access to complete, accurate patient care data; therefore, their interest in CPRs is likely to be high. For example, the Agency for Health Care Policy and Research (AHCPR) is charged to develop uniform definitions of data to be collected and used in describing a patient's clinical and functional status; it also supports the development of common reporting formats and linkages for such data and of standards to ensure data security, confidentiality, accuracy, and maintenance (U.S. Congress, 1989). These activities support or would be supported by CPR implementation.

The research institutes of the National Institutes of Health (NIH) are viewed as stakeholders who would benefit from improved patient data. Within NIH, the National Library of Medicine (NLM) is in a strong position to support CPR development directly through its medical informatics program and its work on the Uniform Medical Language System (UMLS). Further, MEDLINE, HEALTH, and other on-line databases of the NLM's MEDLARS (Medical Literature and Retrieval Systems) are valuable resources for health care professionals that could be made available through CPR workstations.

The Centers for Disease Control (CDC) and the FDA could each benefit from the implementation of CPR systems in two ways. First, CPR implementation would likely improve patient data for epidemiological research.

---

[10]These agencies include the Agency for Health Care Policy and Research, the Centers for Disease Control (including the National Center for Health Statistics), the Food and Drug Administration, the Health Resources and Services Administration, the Indian Health Service, and the National Institutes of Health (including the National Library of Medicine).

Second, direct (i.e., electronic) reporting of events in which these agencies are interested could improve their public health and regulatory activities. Examples of crucial data include occurrences of tracked diseases and information about adverse events related to pharmaceuticals and medical devices.

The Health Resources and Services Administration (HRSA) administers federal support of maternal and child health (MCH) services amounting to more than $525 million a year.[11] MCH programs offer demonstrably more difficult technical and practical barriers to successful implementation of CPRs and CPR systems than do, for instance, traditional hospital inpatient services or physician office-based practices. These obstacles must be recognized, understood, and planned for in the service of improved MCH care. The appendix to this chapter describes how CPRs and CPR systems could support HRSA in meeting its mandate.

The challenges to CPR implementation that are found in MCH programs are by no means unique. For CPRs to be productively and effectively developed and diffused throughout the U.S. health care system, implementers must confront and overcome precisely these kinds of barriers, especially as health care delivery moves more and more into outpatient and nontraditional settings and as it confronts complex "socioclinical" issues related to disadvantaged and underserved populations. Thus, the MCH arena should be seen as a particularly fruitful area in which to design, test, and implement practical computer-based systems for the 1990s.

The Health Care Financing Administration (HCFA) is responsible for administering the Medicare program and the federal portion of Medicaid. Because of the magnitude, scope, and complexity of these programs, HCFA has considerable motivation to improve the efficiency of claims processing, to assess the effectiveness and appropriateness of medical interventions, and to monitor the quality of care rendered. The agency is currently developing a computer-based patient record abstracting system, the Uniform Clinical

---

[11]HRSA uses two main types of funding. The majority of support is awarded to state health agencies through MCH block grants that are intended to enable states to ensure access to maternal and child health services for low-income individuals and individuals who live in areas of limited health resources. The purposes to which these funds can be put are quite broad—ranging from reducing infant mortality and the incidence of preventable diseases to improving the rates of use of diagnostic and therapeutic services.

Most of the remainder of MCH appropriations is disbursed through awards called special projects of regional and national significance (SPRANS). These programs can involve MCH research, training, and projects related to genetic disease testing and counseling and to diagnosis and treatment of hemophilia. More recently, amendments to Title V of the Social Security Act have directed that some funds be used specifically for newborn screening and for child health demonstration projects.

Data Set (UCDS), to improve the efficiency of the Medicare peer review organizations (PROs; Krakauer, 1990). At present, the UCDS must be abstracted manually from hospital charts of Medicare patients; CPR systems would improve the efficiency of collecting these necessary data.

The HCFA Bureau of Program Operations engages in three activities that would benefit from widespread CPR technology. First, the bureau is trying to promote submission of claims by electronic media. Second, it is developing a so-called Common Working File, in which all claims for all kinds of services will be located and accessible upon inquiry. Third, it is seeking to develop a capability for real-time cooperation with PROs that will allow on-line authorization of services.

The Omnibus Budget Reconciliation Act of 1990 (Public Law 101-508) provides for the development of prospective and retrospective drug utilization review (DUR) programs by states participating in Medicaid.[12] The act also includes provisions to conduct demonstration projects to evaluate the efficiency and cost-effectiveness of prospective DURs in patient counseling and reducing costs. Such demonstration projects, which would be overseen by HCFA, are likely to address issues of interest to CPR developers and could support CPR development efforts.

As noted in Chapter 3, the Departments of Defense (DoD) and Veterans Affairs (VA) have installed integrated medical information systems in numerous hospitals (GAO, 1988) and are actively engaged in developing and implementing components of a CPR. Widespread use of CPR systems can be expected to benefit both departments by expanding the availability of technology to meet patient care, research, and education needs. For example, with the CPR, the VA can improve its ability to coordinate health care services provided to veterans in both VA and non-VA settings. The

---

[12]*Drug utilization review* (DUR) is a formal program for comparing data on drug use against explicit, prospective standards and, as necessary, introducing remedial strategies to achieve some desired end. Three primary objectives of DUR are (1) improving quality of care, (2) conserving drug funding resources and controlling individual expenditures, and (3) maintaining program integrity (i.e., controlling fraud and benefit abuse). *Retrospective DUR* is a systematic process that involves selection, review, analysis, and interpretation of drug use data that are collected and analyzed after events occur. Retrospective DUR is used to identify drug utilization trends that warrant further education of practitioners and patients; it also highlights areas of system abuse that might call for more extensive peer-level review and provides mechanisms for evaluation and modification of program criteria and standards. *Prospective DUR* refers to systems that are designed to influence drug prescribing, dispensing, or use in a real-time environment. Implementation of such a system requires that a health care professional with patient care responsibilities have sufficiently detailed information regarding a patient's medical condition, drug use profile, and history to make an informed decision regarding new or renewed drug use (Norris, 1991).

affiliation of VA medical systems with academic medical centers can be enhanced by providing consistency and flexibility for health care professionals at these dispersed sites, thus facilitating collaboration among affiliated institutions.

Although these departments have accomplished a great deal with respect to components of CPR systems, their primary mandate is not patient care. Thus, they cannot be expected to assume primary responsibility for leading CPR development throughout the health care field. Such large health care provider systems, however, can have a great deal of influence on what is developed and produced by vendors.

CONGRESS The potential for Congress to foster CPR development and implementation is great, but its present level of interest in such a course is unclear. Certainly, as evident from the IOM studies on quality assurance in Medicare (IOM, 1990a) and clinical practice guidelines (IOM, 1990b), Congress has expressed a desire to improve the quality of health care.[13] Managing costs remains a critical issue, as is well illustrated by the work of the Physician Payment Review Commission (Lee et al., 1989) and the Prospective Payment Assessment Commission (ProPAC, 1990). Congress is also concerned about improving the quality and availability of health care data for research, a concern reflected in the establishment of AHCPR in late 1989.

Despite Congress's activities on behalf of improved health care, some obstacles to strong congressional support of CPR development may arise. For example, having allocated new monies to some of the efforts noted above, particularly certain parts of the AHCPR mandate, Congress may not see a need for additional specific support to improve patient records. That is, it may believe these problems are being addressed through existing mechanisms. Further, Congress may be especially concerned about the issue of privacy.

In the committee's judgment, better patient records are essential to achieving Congress's health care objectives. Consequently, the central role of the CPR in improving patient records and enhancing quality of care, in managing costs, in facilitating Medicare claims processing, and in improving available data for clinical and health services research must be made clear. Further, CPR advocates must seek to convince key members of Congress that through technological capabilities and legal remedies, CPR systems will bring about a net gain in protecting privacy compared with current record-keeping systems.

---

[13]More recent evidence of Congress's interest in the quality of health care appears in the form of H.R. 1565, which was introduced in the House of Representatives on March 21, 1991. This bill is intended to increase access to health care and to affordable health insurance, as well as to improve health care quality and contain costs.

States

State governments face issues similar to those of the federal government in that they devote significant percentages of their budgets to health care and are concerned about health care quality, cost, and access for their citizens. States have also been fertile grounds for progressive policymaking and legislation. They have played important roles in developing regional databases to monitor quality, manage costs, and assess clinical effectiveness.[14] State governments, cabinet-level health officers, and groups such as the National Conference of State Legislators, Council of State Governments, Association of State and Territorial Health Officials, and National Association of Health Data Organizations could provide a regional perspective in national CPR efforts. In addition, states would be likely candidates for pilot regional studies or experimental prototypes.

Universities and Professional Schools

CPR systems offer several advantages to universities. For example, universities whose professional schools (i.e., schools of medicine, nursing, and dentistry) are involved in clinical research can benefit from the improved data likely to be available for analysis. Furthermore, CPR systems may give the schools a means of disseminating their results for application in clinical practice. (These benefits are likely to accrue to independent research centers as well.)

The interest of health professions schools in CPRs may be mixed, however. On the one hand, faculty members' concerns about threats to their expertise and professional roles might prompt negative reactions to the CPR. On the other hand, individuals in academic or research settings might be

---

[14]The following descriptions are examples of the types of state activities already in progress (National Association of Health Data Organizations, 1988).

In 1977 New York established the Statewide Planning and Research Cooperative System (SPARCS), a public-private effort that provides a unified data system to gather information throughout the state regarding all hospital stays. SPARCS is a major management tool for assisting hospitals, agencies, and other organizations with decision making regarding the financing, planning, and monitoring of inpatient hospital services.

In 1985 the General Assembly of Colorado established the Colorado Health Data Commission to collect, analyze, and disseminate data as a way to encourage competition and informed decision making.

In 1986 the Pennsylvania Health Care Cost Containment Council was established through an act that mandates health care utilization and cost data collection and dissemination. Its central purpose is to increase purchaser and consumer knowledge of health care costs and quality.

more innovative and more receptive to change than health care professionals in other types of settings.

Through the training of health care professionals (including continuing education), professional schools can both shape attitudes toward and provide the skills for using CPRs. Moreover, to the extent that professional schools influence the agenda of researchers (by providing space and support), they can foster the development of CPR systems. Some schools also now serve as centers of medical informatics training and of continuing research in medical informatics.

The NLM supports 11 institutions in efforts to develop prototypes of an Integrated Academic Information Management System (IAIMS). The objective of these projects is to "develop the institutional information infrastructure that permits individuals to access information they need for their clinical or research work from any computer terminal wherever and whenever it is needed" (NAS, 1989). These projects may become models for linking the many departments of academic health and medical centers, including other departments in parent universities (e.g., economics, law, sociology) that have a role to play in clinical and health services research. IAIMS sites may also provide an infrastructure on which to base selected pilot CPR demonstration projects.

Standard-setting Organizations

Two kinds of standard-setting organizations are potential CPR change agents. The first is those groups that are developing standards for health care information systems, primarily in the areas of communication protocols and the characteristics of information collection and use. Among these organizations are the Institute of Electrical and Electronics Engineers (IEEE), the American Society for Testing Materials (ASTM), and the International Standards Organization (ISO). The second kind of standard-setting group comprises various health care accreditation organizations, such as the Joint Commission on Accreditation of Healthcare Organizations, the National Committee on Quality Assurance, and the National League of Nursing. Their role may be to foster CPR development, acquisition, and use by setting standards for accreditation that are most effectively met through CPR systems.

Vendors

CPR system vendors are likely to support development if the projected demand for CPR technology seems sufficient to recoup investment and marketing costs. As discussed earlier, however, vendors are uncertain about the willingness of health care providers to purchase CPR systems. Users or other change agents (such as Congress) may need to provide incentives for a greater or more certain CPR market before vendors can be expected to invest major sums for research, development, or marketing.

Activities and Resources Critical to CPR Development

In light of the various barriers to CPR development, the interest and resources of change agents, and the concerns of stakeholders, the committee identified eight critical activities that will help to advance CPR development: (1) identification and understanding of CPR design requirements; (2) development of standards; (3) CPR and CPR systems research and development; (4) demonstrations of effectiveness, costs, and benefits of CPR systems; (5) reduction of legal constraints for CPR uses as well as enhancement of legal protection for patients; (6) coordination of resources and support for CPR development and diffusion; (7) coordination of information and resources for secondary patient record databases; and (8) education and training of developers and users.

Dedicated resources and improved organization must be provided to accomplish these activities. Resources can take the form of funding, expertise, and equipment. Without adequate funding, however, the other kinds of resources are unlikely to be available. Funding is required to support standard setting, research, demonstrations, review of legal issues, information coordination, education, and a user-developer forum.

Potential sources of funding include federal and state governments, vendors of CPR systems, and private foundations. The committee believes that funding for CPR development should be a governmental priority because the CPR is essential to achieving a variety of ends desired by government (e.g., improved patient care and research). The budget deficits faced by federal and state governments, however, may make the infusion of significant new funds difficult. CPR vendors may be willing to contribute some funds but probably not enough to support all needed activities. Vendors may be more likely to contribute when uncertainty regarding the market for CPR systems has been reduced. Foundations and other groups in the private sector that support health-related research and educational activities may also be an important, indeed, necessary source of funding; again, however, the sums available from this source will not be sufficient to support the entire task envisioned by the committee. Purchasers of systems are unlikely to provide funding for development efforts. They may be willing, however, to contribute in-kind support, for instance, through their participation in demonstration projects.

Substantial levels of resources are already devoted to CPR system development, and this suggests that a major effort should be made to avoid duplication of effort and to build on expertise that has already been developed. The need is great to coordinate CPR-related activities, enhance collaboration, and eliminate potential inefficiencies in the development process. Experience gained from working with currently available data is likely to benefit CPR development. The needs of secondary patient record users may be better met in the interim (i.e., until CPR systems are widely used) through enhancements to existing databases—similar to the approach AHCPR is currently pursuing for research.

Organizational Structure

Health care providers spend large amounts of money on computer and software systems that may not meet their needs today and that will not meet their needs tomorrow.[15] Complete, accurate, accessible patient care data are needed now for clinical care and research. The current combination of private sector, public, and voluntary efforts cannot adequately address the many issues that affect and are related to CPR development and diffusion. Progress is essential on several fronts: coordinating existing and new activities; maximizing public funding; strengthening voluntary efforts (e.g., standard setting); developing a national consensus; and establishing a framework for local efforts.

No one organization currently has the mandate and resources necessary to provide leadership for the CPR effort. Further, the committee concluded that the complexity and importance of the task required an organization dedicated to the CPR mission—such an arrangement would be more likely to foster progress than ad hoc efforts by a number of organizations. Therefore, an initiative should be mounted to create the necessary organizational apparatus, identify and accumulate resources, and pursue the activities noted earlier. This initiative could involve either a new organization created for this purpose or an existing organization that could be given an expanded mission. The organization's fundamental goal would be to facilitate endeavors that improve the flow of information and reduce uncertainty so that a true market for CPRs and CPR systems could function.

Some of these activities are under way, but they are not coordinated with other CPR or CPR-related ventures. Moreover, existing efforts lack authority and national attention. There is also no established mechanism for setting priorities for CPR development or for representing CPR interests on an ongoing basis. The committee believes that the establishment of a formal leadership role is essential for CPR implementation success.

The committee further believes that this leadership role should be established in an organization with the following mission:

---

[15]Nonfederal hospitals in the United States spend more than $5 billion per year on computing-related products and services (Booz-Allen and Hamilton, 1990).

• Support the effective, efficient use of computer-based patient information in patient care, health care policymaking, clinical research, health care financing, and continuous quality improvement.
• Educate change agents and stakeholders (including the general public and health care professionals) about the value of computer-based patient data in improving patient care.
• Foster the CPR as the primary vehicle for collecting patient data.
• Promote the development and use of standards for CPR security and data content, structures, and vocabulary.

Specific steps the organization should take to achieve this mission include the following:

• Establish a forum for CPR users and developers to address such issues as definition of CPR functions and content.
• Facilitate data and security standards setting and endorse such standards.
• Promote CPR data transmission through national high-speed networks by representing the biomedical community in planning for such networks.
• Address legal issues related to CPRs and CPR systems.
• Develop mechanisms for sharing the costs of acquiring and operating CPR systems among all users of CPR data.
• Define priorities and criteria for CPR demonstration projects that could be used by federal agencies, private foundations, and health care provider institutions.
• Conduct workshops and conferences to educate health care professionals and policymakers.
• Explore the need for a clearinghouse or data center for secondary CPR information.

Given the mission and objectives outlined above, the committee concluded that any organization leading the effort to advance the implementation of CPRs should have several key attributes. First, it should be national in scope. Second, it should have authority to make and implement decisions. Third, it should represent all CPR users, as well as CPR developers. Fourth, it must have sufficient visibility and influence to be able to achieve measurable progress within a relatively short time. Three to five years was seen as a reasonable time frame for initial headway to be made.

The committee had particular concerns about the feasibility of establishing and operating such an organization. To clarify the issues further, it examined several organizational models in terms of the need for and ability to secure funding, receive a mandate, and gain acceptance. The three main options explored by the committee were a purely governmental (federal) effort, a purely private sector entity, and some form of a public-private commission, consortium, council, or institute. The advantages and disadvantages of these options are discussed below.[16]

Federal Agency

There are several advantages to a federally based CPR development effort. In general, a federal initiative associated with an existing agency has implied authority and power, as well as lower start-up and operating costs than would be incurred for a newly created, freestanding organization. Moreover, congressional support is likely to be stronger if the CPR effort is closely linked to federal efforts that are already under way. In addition, staff would not need to spend time raising funds as would be necessary for a private sector effort.

A federal agency would have less independence than a private sector organization, however, and would face possible limitations from bureaucratic policies and procedures. Thus, greater potential for innovation might exist in the private sector. Another disadvantage to locating leadership for CPR development within the federal government is the potential for health care providers to see such efforts as too closely aligned with government and therefore open to excessive regulation and intrusiveness. Finally, such an approach must rely on receiving a mandate and funding, which could make start-up time for federal efforts longer than for a private organization.

Within DHHS, several agencies might be considered. First, the Office of the Assistant Secretary for Planning and Evaluation (ASPE) might be able to bridge the gaps among various agencies and programs in DHHS. It would be unlikely, however, to gather the resources and expertise required to mount an effort of the magnitude envisioned by this report.

AHCPR has functions quite consistent with the objectives of the leadership entity proposed by the committee, although these functions are not its primary responsibilities. Currently, AHCPR does not have the resources to undertake a CPR implementation project, but if such funding were forthcoming it could, over time, assume a more significant role. One drawback, however, is that such an effort might be seen as possibly undermining the agency's main mission—that is, support of health services, outcomes, and effectiveness research and the development of clinical practice guidelines.

HCFA has a substantial interest in the CPR for both operational and quality improvement reasons. Although HCFA would be a key beneficiary of widespread CPR implementation and hence likely to want to provide

---

[16]To address this issue fully, the committee organized a one-day workshop in September 1990 to evaluate the feasibility and desirability of alternative organizational models for a CPR organization; AHCPR provided separate funding for the meeting. Workshop participants included representatives of health care professionals, provider institutions, federal agencies, insurers, employers, and private foundations.

critical resources, it may not be the ideal agency to champion patient record development. If HCFA were to lead the CPR effort, health care providers might not be able to separate it from HCFA's other activities, particularly regulation of the Medicare program, cost containment, and related efforts. Providers might resist the CPR development initiative because of a perception that it was intended as a cost-containment mechanism rather than as a way to improve health care delivery.

The Departments of Defense (DoD) and Veterans Affairs (VA) are both making significant investments in comprehensive medical information systems.[17] As a result, they have a great deal of expertise in designing and implementing such systems. These departments do not seem likely candidates for leading a CPR initiative, however, because of their restricted populations and other non-health care responsibilities. In short, no existing federal organization simultaneously has the mandate, mission, credibility, and resources to take on this responsibility.

Private Sector Sponsorship

The committee also considered a private sector, not-for-profit membership organization, similar to the Joint Commission on the Accreditation of Healthcare Organizations, to lead the CPR development effort. A decided advantage to a purely private approach is that the conversion to computer-based records would become something championed by, rather than imposed on, these organizations and their constituents. The active involvement of such organizations might prompt them to provide core funding, and the efforts to secure funding from others might then be more effective. In addition, staff recruitment for a private organization would be facilitated by the broad-based support the organization would receive from national health care groups.

This strategy has its limitations, however. Most important is that such an organization would lack the power and authority implicit in a governmental entity. Further, federal funding could be difficult to obtain unless key agencies played a major role in the organization's activities.

Public-Private Commission or Consortium

In theory, a public-private organization would offer the advantage of involving and being able to draw on funding and personnel resources from

---

[17]DoD is acquiring the Composite Health Care System for installation in its 167 hospitals and nearly 600 clinics. The costs for full deployment of this system are expected to be $1.6 billion. The VA is installing the Decentralized Hospital Computer System to support its 172 hospitals and 358 outpatient facilities. The VA estimates that this system as currently defined will cost $925 million (GAO, 1988, 1990).

both sectors. Furthermore, because the problems with patient records affect both public and private organizations, acceptance of a solution would be more likely if both sectors were involved in the decision-making process.

The drawbacks of a public-private entity should not be underestimated, however. Managing the diverse interests that would be represented in such an organization presents a major challenge. Certain federal agencies already have charters that would overlap the charge to such an organization. In addition, a purely private sector organization might offer more entrepreneurial agility than a hybrid group. Perhaps the biggest drawback of a public-private organization is the inherent instability of such an approach. Lacking a federal mandate and given the less-than-immediate contribution to the profitability of private sector participants concerned with CPR development, a public-private organization may not command sufficient resources and attention to address effectively the barriers to CPRs and CPR systems.

Preferred Approach

The committee recognizes that the federal sector has considerable resources (including authority and knowledge) to influence CPR development. For example, HCFA can establish reimbursement mechanisms that reward providers who submit insurance claims generated by CPR systems. AHCPR is expressly mandated to improve patient data for research. The VA and DoD have gained considerable experience in CPR development and implementation. NLM has made significant contributions to the management of medical knowledge for practitioners.

Nevertheless, several factors militate against a purely federal approach. First, the resources, potential change agents, and stakeholders that must be coordinated or engaged in CPR development are present in both the public and private sectors. Thus, a structure is needed that can draw from both sectors. Second, the committee believes that routine use of the CPR can be achieved most efficiently through a collaborative process that develops consensus on key issues (e.g., data and security standards, the minimum content of CPR systems) yet allows flexibility at the local level to foster innovation in the development and use of CPRs.

Third, the committee believes that patient care should be the primary focus of CPR development and implementation. Practitioner use of CPR systems requires that the systems meet practitioner needs, and only if practitioners are willing to use CPR systems to capture data and to secure assistance in clinical decision making can the benefits of CPRs for moderating costs and conducting research be realized. It is essential that practitioners view the CPR as a valuable resource for improving patient care. Thus, CPR efforts must involve health care providers as well as federal agencies.

CPR design should not be driven solely by governmental objectives—for example, those embodied in the cost-containment and health outcomes research missions of HCFA and AHCPR, respectively. Although those agencies are likely to have significant interest in CPR development, their primary mission is not patient care.

The committee concluded that a public-private approach would be optimal in the long run and, as elaborated in Chapter 5, proposes the establishment of a Computer-based Patient Record Institute (CPRI). It was also of the view that the potential base of funding in the private sector is not sufficiently solid to provide adequate support for a new organization at this time. This judgment was founded on its review of the history of CPR development and on a poll of the participants at the workshop noted earlier. As a result, the committee also concluded that a federally initiated and funded approach would be most appropriate for necessary interim activities.

Immediate action is needed to advance CPR efforts and to lay the groundwork for an organization such as the CPRI that would ultimately coordinate the necessary infrastructure for a national CPR system. Many of the barriers to CPR implementation relate to lack of information; part of the interim effort thus should focus on education and evaluation. Standards development and representation of the interests of health care in the national high-speed computer network discussed earlier should also be given high-priority attention. The overall goal of such efforts would be, within five years, to turn over operational issues to a public-private organization that is supported mainly by its members.

The committee noted that if the private sector failed to support CPR efforts adequately, the federal government might still be sufficiently motivated to advance the CPR unilaterally. Long-term dominance by the federal government in this area could result in an approach that was more regulatory and bureaucratic than collaborative and innovative. To preclude such an eventuality, the committee placed special importance on joint public and private sector progress.

This approach is consistent with the recent General Accounting Office report on automated medical records (GAO, 1991), which made two recommendations to the secretary of Health and Human Services. First, as part of DHHS's mandate to conduct research on outcomes of health care services, the secretary should "direct the Public Health Service, through its Agency for Health Care Policy and Research, to support the exploration of ways in which automated medical records can be used to more effectively and efficiently provide data for outcomes research" (GAO, 1991:26). Second, as part of the effort to support outcomes research, the secretary should "develop a plan and budget for consideration by the Congress, to bring about the greater use of automated medical records" (GAO, 1991:26). Specific elements of such a plan could include "a national forum that sets goals for automating medical information, addresses individual and organizational concerns with automated records, and identifies incentives to induce health care organizations to increase their use of automation" (GAO, 1991:26).

Specific Steps for Change Agents

The challenges of developing affordable CPR systems that are acceptable to users and of achieving widespread use of such systems within a decade should not be underestimated or understated. Much of the progress toward these goals is likely to occur incrementally over time and across the country. The CPRI can play an important role in tracking progress and directing future efforts, but significant contributions to CPR development and implementation can and must be made by individuals and groups other than the CPRI. A great deal of work can be accomplished at the regional, local, and institutional levels in preparation for CPR implementation.

• As discussed earlier in this chapter, health care professionals could support development and implementation by helping to plan and conduct research or demonstrations of CPR systems. Involvement of all kinds of CPR users is needed—especially practitioners as the primary source of data—to design systems that will meet their requirements.

• Professional societies could implement formal education and awareness programs as part of their membership mailings and annual meetings. They could also support conferences at which CPR users could share experiences, report on useful experiments in various settings, and meet with other professional disciplines to discuss data and function needs.

• Purchasers of CPR systems could actively seek systems that are able to meet basic data-exchange and security standards and offer sufficient capacity to evolve over time.

• Insurers could offer incentives (e.g., faster payment of claims) for data that are provided in electronic form.

• Health care business coalitions, chambers of commerce, and major employers could all support CPR development and implementation efforts by supporting research and pilot demonstrations as well as by developing relationships with insurers and health care provider institutions that use or support CPR systems.

• Federal agencies could provide substantial funding for research and development and support standards development through funding or regulatory mandate.

• States could serve as candidates for pilot regional studies or experimental prototypes.

• Health care accreditation organizations could foster CPR development, acquisition, and use by setting standards for accreditation that are most effectively met through CPR systems.

• In their training of health care professionals (including continuing education), professional schools could both shape attitudes toward and provide the skills for using CPRs. They could also foster the development of CPR systems to the extent that the agenda of researchers is influenced by the schools' provision of space and support.

• Researchers could study the costs and benefits of CPR systems, at both micro and macro levels, including the impact of CPR systems on the quality and costs of care.

• State agencies, hospital associations, and local professional groups could establish working groups to develop a common understanding and vision of how CPRs could support their health care environment and to identify the elements of local and regional infrastructure needed to support future CPRs. Working groups could study the relationships among referring physicians and among other providers to understand their entire system of health care. They could also define needed data elements, educate local health care professionals on health care information management issues, and monitor progress in the development of standards for security and data exchange.

SUMMARY

In addition to technological advances, successful implementation of CPR systems requires elimination of the barriers to development and diffusion. It also requires that the concerns of stakeholders be addressed and that potential change agents be engaged.

Many impediments to the CPR arise from a lack of awareness and understanding of CPRs and their capabilities. System purchasers and users lack adequate information about the benefits and costs of CPRs. In particular, developers and vendors require more specific information about what users want from systems and what price providers would be willing to pay for systems that meet their needs. Activities aimed at improving (e.g., demonstration projects) and disseminating (e.g., education programs) available information about CPR systems constitute an important step for CPR implementation.

Other impediments arise from the lack of an infrastructure to support CPR development and diffusion. Such an infrastructure comprises standards for communication of data (i.e., vocabulary control and data format standards); laws and regulations that protect patient privacy but do not inhibit transfer of information to legitimate users of data outside the clinical setting; experts trained in the development and use of CPR systems; institutional, local, regional, and national networks for transmitting CPR data; reimbursement mechanisms that pay for the costs of producing improved patient care information; and a management structure (i.e., an organization) for setting priorities, garnering and allocating resources, and coordinating activities. Removal of these impediments is essential to the timely development and implementation of CPR systems.

REFERENCES

Agranoff, M. H. 1989. Curb on technology: Liability for failure to protect computerized data against unauthorized access. *Computer and High Technology Law Journal* 5:263-320.

Amatayakul, M., and M. J. Wogan. 1989. Fundamental considerations related to the Institute of Medicine Patient Record Project. Paper prepared for the Institute of Medicine Committee on Improving Patient Records in Response to Increasing Functional Requirements and Technological Advances.

Anderson, J. G., and S. J. Jay. 1987. The diffusion of computer applications in medical settings. Pp. 3-7 in *Use and Impact of Computers in Clinical Medicine*, ed. J. G. Anderson and S. J. Jay. New York: Springer-Verlag.

Anderson, J. G., S. J. Jay, H. M. Schweer, M. A. Anderson, and D. Kassing. 1987. Physician communication networks and the adoption and utilization of computer applications in medicine. Pp. 185-199 in *Use and Impact of Computers in Clinical Medicine*, ed. J. G. Anderson and S. J. Jay. New York: Springer-Verlag.

Banta, H. D. 1987. Embracing or rejecting innovations: Clinical diffusion of health care technology. Pp. 132-160 in *Use and Impact of Computers in Clinical Medicine*, ed. J. G. Anderson and S. J. Jay. New York: Springer-Verlag.

Blendon, R. J. 1988. The public's view of the future of health care. *Journal of the American Medical Association* 250:3587-3593.

Booz-Allen and Hamilton. 1990. Response to the Strategy and Implementation Subcommittee Report to the Institute of Medicine Committee on Improving the Patient Record. Bethesda, Md.

Bradbury, A. 1990. Computerized medical records: The need for a standard. *Journal of the American Medical Association* 61:25-35.

Brannigan, V. M., and R. E. Dayhoff. 1986. Medical informatics: The revolution in law, technology, and medicine. *Journal of Legal Medicine* 7:1-53.

Bronzino, J. D., V. H. Smith, and M. L. Wade. 1990. *Medical Technology and Society: An Interdisciplinary Perspective*. New York: McGraw-Hill Publishing Company.

Clepper, P. 1991. Communication to committee. National Library of Medicine, Bethesda, Md.

Denis, S., and Y. Poullet. 1990. Questions of liability in the provision of information services. *Online Review* 14:21-32.

Dowling, A. F. 1987. Do hospital staff interfere with computer system implementation? Pp. 302-317 in *Use and Impact of Computers in Clinical Medicine*, ed. J. G. Anderson and S. J. Jay. New York: Springer-Verlag.

Food and Drug Administration. 1989. Draft Policy for the Regulation of Computer Products (photocopy). Washington, D.C.

Gabrieli, E. R., and G. Murphy. 1990. Computerized medical records. *Journal of the American Medical Association* 61:26-31.

GAO (General Accounting Office). 1987. ADP Systems: Examinations of Non-federal Hospital Information Systems. IMTEX-87-21. Washington, D.C. June.

GAO. 1988. Use of Information Technology in Hospitals. Statement of Melroy D. Quasney, Associate Director, Information Management and Technology Division, before the Subcommittee on Education and Health, Joint Economic Committee. T-IMTEC-88-4. Washington, D.C. May 24.

GAO. 1990. Defense's Acquisition of the Composite Health Care System. Statement of Daniel C. White, Special Assistant to the Assistant Comptroller General, before the Subcommittee on Military Personnel and Compensation, Committee on Armed Services, U.S. House of Representatives. T-IMTEC-90-04. March 15.

GAO. 1991. *Medical ADP Systems: Automated Medical Records Hold Promise to Improve Patient Care.* Washington, D.C.

Gould, S. 1990a. *CRS Issue Brief: Building the National Research and Education Network.* Washington, D.C.: Library of Congress.

Gould, S. 1990b. *CRS Report for Congress: The Federal Research Internet and the National Research and Education Network. Prospects for the 1990s.* Washington, D.C.: Library of Congress.

Hard, R. 1990. Computers help keep patient files confidential. *Hospitals* 179:49-50.

Henley, R. R., and G. Wiederhold. 1975. An Analysis of Automated Ambulatory Care Medical Record Systems [AARMS]: Findings. AARMS Study Group, University of California, San Francisco. June.

IOM (Institute of Medicine). 1990a. *Clinical Practice Guidelines: Directions for a New Program*, ed. M. J. Field and K. N. Lohr. Washington, D.C.: National Academy Press.

IOM. 1990b. *Medicare: A Strategy for Quality Assurance*, vols. 1 and 2, ed. K. N. Lohr. Washington, D.C.: National Academy Press.

Kaplan, B. 1987. The influence of medical values and practices on medical computer applications. Pp. 39-50 in *Use and Impact of Computers in Clinical Medicine*, ed. J. G. Anderson and S. J. Jay. New York: Springer-Verlag.

Koster, A., F. L. Waterstraat, and N. Sondak. 1987. Automated and ambulatory record systems: A comparative costs analysis. *Journal of the American Medical Record Association* 58:26-31.

Krakauer, H. 1990. The uniform clinical data set. Pp. 120-133 in *Effectiveness and Outcomes in Health Care*, ed. K. A. Heithoff and K. N. Lohr. Washington, D.C.: National Academy Press.

Lee, P. R., P. B. Ginsburg, L. R. LeRoy, and G. T. Hammons. 1989. The Physician Payment Review Commission report to Congress. *Journal of the American Medical Association* 261:2382-2388.

Lindberg, D. A. B. 1970. A statewide medical information system. *Computers and Biomedical Research* 3:453-463.

Lindberg, D. A. B. 1979. The development and diffusion of a medical technology: Medical information systems. Pp. 201-239 in *Medical Technology and the Health Care System: A Study of the Diffusion of Equipment-Embodied Technology.* Washington, D.C.: National Academy of Sciences.

Lindberg, D. A. B., and B. L. Humphreys. 1990. The Unified Medical Language System and the Automated Patient Record. Paper prepared for the Institute of

Medicine Committee on Improving Patient Records in Response to Increasing Functional Requirements and Technological Advances.

Masys, D. R. 1990. Of codes and keywords: Standards for biomedical nomenclature. *Academic Medicine* 65:627-629.

McDonald, C. J., and W. E. Hammond. 1989. Standard format for electronic transfer of clinical data. *Annals of Internal Medicine* 110:333-335.

McDonald, C. J., and W. M. Tierney. 1988. Computer-stored medical records: Their future role in medical practice. *Journal of the American Medical Association* 259:3433-3440.

Metzger, M. C. 1988. Legal implications of computer-aided medical diagnosis. *Journal of Legal Medicine* 9:313-328.

NAS (National Academy of Sciences). 1979. *Medical Technology and the Health Care System: A Study of the Diffusion of Equipment-Embodied Technology.* Washington, D.C.: National Academy of Sciences.

NAS. 1989. *Information Technology and the Conduct of Research: The Users' View.* Washington, D.C.: National Academy Press.

National Association of Health Data Organizations (NAHDO). 1988. *NAHDO Resource Manual.* Washington, D.C. March.

National Center for Health Statistics. 1990. *The National Committee on Vital and Health Statistics, 1989.* Hyattsville, Md.

National Conference of Commissioners on Uniform State Laws. 1986. *Uniform Health-Care Information Act.* Chicago, Ill.

National Science Foundation. 1990. Report on Selected Congressional Activities. 101st Cong., 2d sess. NSB-90-117. Washington, D.C.: Office of Legislative and Public Affairs. December.

Norris, J. 1991. Communication to committee. Drug Utilization Review and Point of Sale Systems. Hill and Knowlton, Waltham, Mass. March.

NRC (National Research Council). 1991. *Computers at Risk: Safe Computing in the Information Age.* Washington, D.C.: National Academy Press.

OTA (Office of Technology Assessment). 1977. *Policy Implications of Medical Information Systems.* OTA-H-56. Washington, D.C.: U.S. Government Printing Office.

Peck, R. S. 1984. Extending the constitutional right to privacy in the new technological age. *Hofstra Law Review* 12:893-912.

Privacy Protection Study Commission. 1977. *Personal Privacy in an Information Society.* Washington, D.C.: U.S. Government Printing Office.

ProPAC (Prospective Payment Assessment Commission). 1990. *Medicare Prospective Payment and the American Health Care System: Report to Congress.* Washingon, D.C. June.

Rogers, E. M. 1987. Diffusion of innovations: An overview. Pp. 113-131 in *Use and Impact of Computers in Clinical Medicine,* ed. J. G. Anderson and S. G. Jay. New York: Springer-Verlag.

Teach, R. L., and E. H. Shortliffe. 1981. An analysis of physician attitudes regarding computer-based clinical consultation systems. *Computers and Biomedical Research* 14:542-558.

U.S. Congress. 1989. *Congressional Record,* vol. 135, no. 165, pt. 3. November 21.

Washington Business Group on Health. 1989. *Fostering Uniformity for Health Care Assessment Data Gathering.* Washington, D.C.

Westin, A. F. 1976. *Computers, Health Records and Citizen Rights.* National Bureau of Standards Monograph 157. Washington, D.C.: U.S. Government Printing Office.

Willick, M. S. 1986. Professional malpractice and the unauthorized practice of professions: Some legal and ethical aspects of the use of computers as decision-aids. *Rutgers Computer and Technology Law Journal* 12:1-32.

Young, D. W. 1987. What makes doctors use computers? Discussion paper. Pp. 8-14 in *Use and Impact of Computers in Clinical Medicine*, ed. J. G. Anderson and S. J. Jay. New York: Springer-Verlag.

APPENDIX: MATERNAL AND CHILD HEALTH CARE AND COMPUTER-BASED PATIENT RECORDS

As discussed in Chapter 3, much of the progress to date in implementing CPRs and CPR systems has occurred in hospitals and large multispecialty practices, particularly in health maintenance organizations. To be successful, however, CPRs and the larger computer-based systems in which they function must be useful and practical for many other types of providers, including, for instance, community-based clinics and other outpatient facilities serving either primary care or special health care needs. In this category might fall services to disadvantaged populations such as those eligible for maternal and child health care through Title V of the Social Security Act.

The area of maternal and child health (MCH), both generally and as administered by the Health Resources and Services Administration (HRSA) in support of the Title V mandate, poses particularly interesting challenges and opportunities for CPRs and CPR systems. Five topics are briefly discussed here as examples.

First, the challenges involve, among other matters, the capability to *track populations* that typically do not have regular providers of care; that move in and out of eligibility for the services; that move in and out of geographic areas (e.g., states, underserved regions) where the services are provided; and that are in many ways socially, economically, and demographically disadvantaged. In such circumstances, ease of data entry, storage, and transmission of clinical and sociodemographic information takes on special importance. CPRs can maximize these attributes, especially in comparison to traditional paper records that are often institution-specific, fragmented, illegible, and lacking in information related to social support, health education, and similar nonclinical issues. Another important factor in reaching these populations is coordination of care across many different sites. Computer-based systems will facilitate timely, accurate movement of necessary information and collaboration among those delivering both clinical and social services.

Second, MCH programs are expected to reach out to obstetricians, gynecologists, and pediatricians throughout the states, to develop integrated

MCH service delivery programs, to improve home visit programs (including those concerned with case management), to collaborate with inpatient institutions delivering care to children with special health care needs, and to improve services to rural populations. CPR systems should make it easier to achieve these objectives by making *clinical and sociodemographic data more readily available even in relatively nontraditional settings.* Certainly the expectation of CPR developers and innovators is that their technologies, when broadly implemented, will offer capabilities far beyond what can be achieved with today's paper medical charts, particularly in terms of longitudinal records in which, for instance, information about immunizations and screening services must be maintained over a considerable period of time.

A third major challenge facing HRSA and its MCH bureau is the required implementation of relatively recent mandates of Title V that call for *development and maintenance of a data and information system.* Part of this system presumably would involve the acquisition of pertinent epidemiological data that can be used by the bureau and others to improve and promote health and prevent disease among mothers, infants, children, and others eligible for MCH block grant services. To the extent that CPRs and CPR systems allow institutional providers and practitioners (e.g., physicians, visiting nurses, clinic staff) to enter data once (and only once) for both clinical and administrative purposes, they will considerably simplify the reporting requirements of these programs. Moreover, the expectation is that CPR systems ultimately will communicate with each other with the aid of a composite clinical data dictionary (CCDD); this means that states, and the providers and clinicians who operate in them, will not need to conform rigidly to a single federal data system in meeting HRSA's reporting requirements (because the federal system itself would be a party to the CCDD).

A fourth way in which the movement toward CPRs and CPR systems may be important for MCH activities concerns the *support of research.* As a general proposition, researchers are more accustomed to the use of computers for data gathering and analysis than are clinicians, so movement toward the implementation of such systems presumably would be regarded as welcome progress by those involved in MCH research. Indeed, one specific aim of research grants in this area is to use automated systems to facilitate the management and delivery of health care for target populations.

One special aspect of the research effort involves infant mortality and Medicaid (Title XIX) services. The secretary of Health and Human Services is expected to develop a national data system for linking vital statistics (birth and death) records with information on Medicaid insurance claims forms. This task clearly lies within the realm of CPR development.

In a related vein, special projects may be mounted to enhance family-centered and community-based health care, both within and across states.

These projects could benefit greatly from a capacity to acquire large amounts of information, locate those data securely in a single site (for analysis and archival purposes), and make them available to properly authorized users for analysis (and perhaps for clinical purposes as well). The collection, storage, maintenance, and use of such information through computer-based systems, rather than through paper records (or paper records secondarily data-entered into computer files), can be expected over the long run to promote more comprehensive and more productive special projects on this and other complex topics (e.g., services to children with serious impairments and handicaps such as spina bifida, debilitating chronic illnesses, or cleft lip and palate).

The fifth point relates more specifically to the *potential value of communication and collaboration across federal agencies.* Several federal departments have already taken steps to design and implement one or more components of a CPR system. Notable among these are the Departments of Defense (DoD) and Veterans Affairs (VA). Both departments have health care delivery responsibilities for distinct, and sometimes quite dispersed, populations that have both traditional primary care needs (e.g., for screening and prevention) and health care problems at least equivalent in complexity and severity to those facing disadvantaged MCH populations. Both departments also have considerable health research programs. Lessons from their efforts to date may prove helpful in planning computer-based systems to serve MCH needs; conversely, issues that arise in planning for and delivering services to disadvantaged MCH populations might be posed to DoD and the VA as a means of bringing difficult technical questions to their attention.

In addition, the Health Care Financing Administration (HCFA) has mounted an interesting effort to develop a "uniform clinical data set"; although it is oriented toward hospital care (and care for the elderly), its developmental history to date offers useful and perhaps cautionary lessons for others attempting to develop clinical data sets and data dictionaries. Certainly it would be important for HCFA developers to understand the special needs and perspectives of a computer-based data set oriented more toward Medicaid than toward Medicare.

Finally, the Agency for Health Care Policy and Research (AHCPR) has a specific congressional mandate to work toward the development of computer databases that will serve broad clinical evaluation purposes. Part of AHCPR's interest has been specifically in computer-based record systems, including the potential for a public, or public-private, entity to undertake many technical, legal, and other tasks related to the establishment of CPRs and CPR systems nationally over the next decade. Because the MCH component of HRSA will have wide concerns about quality of care, outcomes of care, and similar issues, it would seem prudent for HRSA to work together from the outset with a sister Public Health Service agency on many of these subjects.

5

Improving Patient Records:
Conclusions and Recommendations

Computer-based patient records and the systems in which they function are becoming an essential technology for health care in part because the information management challenges faced by health care professionals are increasing daily. Technological progress makes it possible for CPRs and CPR systems to provide total, cost-effective access to more complete, accurate patient care data and to offer improved performance and enhanced functions that can be used to meet those information management challenges. CPRs can play an important role in improving the quality of patient care and strengthening the scientific basis of clinical practice; they can also contribute to the management and moderation of health care costs.

The Institute of Medicine (IOM) study committee believes that the time is right for a major initiative to make CPRs a standard technology in health care within a decade. Achieving this goal within 10 years will require a nationwide effort and a great deal of work. More research and development are needed in several critical areas to ensure that systems meet the needs of patients, practitioners, administrators, third-party payers, researchers, and policymakers. For example, the need to protect patient privacy must be balanced by the need for timely access to data at multiple sites. Systems must offer both considerable flexibility for users and standards required for data transfer and exchange.

CPR implementation will necessitate both organizational and behavioral changes. Organizationally, it will require substantial coordination across the many elements of the pluralistic U.S. health care system. Behaviorally, it will demand that users develop new skills to use CPR systems and to change their documentation behaviors.

BOX 5-1 SUMMARY OF THE RECOMMENDATIONS OF THE INSTITUTE OF MEDICINE COMMITTEE ON IMPROVING THE PATIENT RECORD

The committee recommends the following:

1. Health care professionals and organizations should adopt the computer-based patient record (CPR) as the standard for medical and all other records related to patient care.

2. To accomplish Recommendation 1, the public and private sectors should join in establishing a Computer-based Patient Record Institute (CPRI) to promote and facilitate development, implementation, and dissemination of the CPR.

3. Both the public and private sectors should expand support for the CPR and CPR system implementation through research, development, and demonstration projects. Specifically, the committee recommends that Congress authorize and appropriate funds to implement the research and development agenda outlined herein. The committee further recommends that private foundations and vendors fund programs that support and facilitate this research and development agenda.

4. The CPRI should promulgate uniform national standards for data and security to facilitate implementation of the CPR and its secondary databases.

5. The CPRI should review federal and state laws and regulations for the purpose of proposing and promulgating model legislation and regulations to facilitate the implementation and dissemination of the CPR and its secondary databases and to streamline the CPR and CPR systems.

6. The costs of CPR systems should be shared by those who benefit from the value of the CPR. Specifically, the full costs of implementing and operating CPRs and CPR systems should be factored into reimbursement levels or payment schedules of both public and private sector third-party payers. In addition, users of secondary databases should support the costs of creating such databases.

7. Health care professional schools and organizations should enhance educational programs for students and practitioners in the use of computers, CPRs, and CPR systems for patient care, education, and research.

This chapter summarizes the committee's principal conclusions and presents recommendations for improving patient records (see Box 5-1). These recommendations, to which committee members gave unanimous approval, outline a course to facilitate the transition of health care away from the current paper patient record and toward routine use of the CPR and its supporting CPR system. Specifically, the committee's recommendations recognize the CPR as the standard patient record of the future, provide an organizational framework for overcoming barriers to CPR development and implementation, and identify steps that will advance the use of CPRs and CPR systems.

CONCLUSIONS

Patient records are the primary repository of data in the information-intensive health care industry. Although clinical information is increasingly likely to be computerized, the current, predominant mode for recording patient care data remains the paper record. Paper records have the advantages of being familiar to users and portable; when they are not too large, users can readily browse through them. Paper records, however, have serious, overriding limitations that frequently frustrate users and perpetuate inefficiencies in the health care system. Further, the impact of these limitations is growing as the health care system becomes more complex. Modern patient care requirements have outgrown the paper record.

Quality improvement and cost containment continue to be major concerns for the health care industry. Quality assurance; utilization management; appropriateness, effectiveness, and outcomes assessment; clinical practice guidelines; and value purchasing are all prominent responses to the quality or cost challenges faced by present-day health care. Each of these initiatives increases the legitimate demand for complete, accurate, readily accessible patient data.

Health care professionals today face an unprecedented information explosion as the quantity and complexity of patient data and medical knowledge increase practically daily. Current patient records cannot adequately manage all the information needed for patient care. Paper patient records have not kept and cannot keep pace with the rapidly changing health care system. As a result, they increasingly impede effective decision making throughout the health care sector—from the bedside to the formulation of national health care policy.

Some health care institutions are already applying computer technologies to this information management challenge. In general, however, the diffusion of information management technologies has been slower in health care than in other information-intensive industries. Moreover, the majority of information management applications in the health care sector have focused on financial and administrative rather than clinical data.

In its study, the committee reviewed the needs of patient record users, as well as existing and emerging computer technologies. It concluded that better CPR systems—systems that meet user needs more fully—can be achieved within 10 years. Nevertheless, the committee cautions that merely automating current patient records will perpetuate their deficiencies and will not be sufficient to satisfy emerging user demands. If future patient records are to be an asset in patient care, they must offer broader functions than those provided by the record systems of today.

The future patient record will be a computer-based, multimedia record capable of including free text, high-resolution images, sound (e.g., auscultations), full-motion video, and elaborate coding schemes. CPR systems will offer access (availability, convenience, speed, reliability, and ease of use), quality, security, flexibility, connectivity, and efficiency. In addition, future patient records will provide new functions through links to other databases and decision support tools.

No contemporary clinical information systems are sufficiently comprehensive to be considered full CPR systems. Several existing systems, however, offer prototypes of components of CPR systems.

The committee considers nine technological capabilities to be essential to CPR systems: (1) databases and database management systems, (2) workstations, (3) data acquisition and retrieval, (4) text processing, (5) image processing and storage, (6) data-exchange and vocabulary standards, (7) system communications and network infrastructure, (8) system reliability and security, and (9) linkages to secondary databases.

No new technological breakthroughs are needed to develop robust CPR systems, but some emerging technologies are crucial. Low-cost yet powerful clinical workstations and improved human interface technologies are needed. Voice-recognition systems, high-capacity networks (e.g., fiberoptic), and open-architecture systems will be required to achieve broad adoption of CPR systems. Emerging clipboard-sized computers that accept input through a hand-held stylus may also prove to be a critical development. In addition, CPR diffusion requires development of standards for health care data and greater emphasis on protecting the integrity and confidentiality of CPR data.

Technology is not the only potentially limiting factor in advancing CPR systems; informational, organizational, and behavioral barriers must also be addressed. Barriers to CPR development include development costs and lack of consensus on CPR content. CPR diffusion is adversely affected by the disaggregated health care environment, the complex characteristics of CPR technology, unpredictable user behavior, the high costs of acquiring CPR systems, a lack of adequate networks for transmitting data, a lack of leadership for resolving CPR issues, a lack of training for CPR developers and users, and a variety of legal and social issues.

The committee developed a plan for advancing the development and implementation of CPRs and CPR systems that identifies a broad group of stakeholders who would be affected (both positively and negatively) by CPR system implementation. It also identifies a group of organizations that, in the committee's view, could contribute significantly to such development and implementation. Finally, the plan identifies a series of activities that would advance CPR efforts.

Carrying out these activities will require adequate funding and effective organization. The committee reviewed organizational structures that could be used to provide the necessary framework for coordinating CPR activities. It concluded that no existing organization has the mandate and resources necessary to lead this effort. Thus, the committee believes that a new organization is needed to support CPR development and implementation. The committee proposes a framework for the establishment of such an organization, but it also emphasizes that securing adequate resources for and engaging the appropriate parties in CPR development efforts are more important than the precise structure of the recommended organization.

RECOMMENDATIONS

RECOMMENDATION 1. The committee recommends that health care professionals and organizations adopt the computer-based patient record (CPR) as the standard for medical and all other records related to patient care.

The committee believes that future patient records must be more than a way to store patient data—they must also support the clinical decision process and help improve the quality of patient care. Achieving widespread use of CPRs is a major component of building a national health care information system that can support the provision of integrated health care services across settings and providers of care. Further, widespread use of CPRs would contribute to the collection of patient care data as a national health care resource. Achieving these objectives requires that CPRs be more than automated paper records.

The committee defined the CPR as an electronic patient record (i.e., a repository of health care information about a single patient) that resides in a system specifically designed to support users through availability of complete and accurate data, alerts, reminders, clinical decision support systems, links to medical knowledge, and other aids. Further, the committee identified 12 attributes that comprehensive CPRs and CPR systems possess.

1. The CPR contains a problem list that clearly delineates the patient's clinical problems and the current status of each (e.g., the primary illness is worsening, stable, or improving).

2. The CPR encourages and supports the systematic measurement and recording of the patient's health status and functional level to promote more precise and routine assessment of the outcomes of patient care.

3. The CPR states the logical basis for all diagnoses or conclusions as a means of documenting the clinical rationale for decisions about the management of the patient's care. (This documentation should enhance use of a scientific approach in clinical practice and assist the evolution of a firmer foundation for clinical knowledge.)

4. The CPR can be linked with other clinical records of a patient—from various settings and time periods—to provide a longitudinal (i.e., lifelong) record of events that may have influenced a person's health.

5. The CPR system addresses patient data confidentiality comprehensively—in particular, ensuring that the CPR is accessible only to authorized individuals. (Although absolute confidentiality cannot be guaranteed in any system, every possible practical and cost-effective measure should be taken to secure CPRs and CPR systems from unauthorized access or abuse.)

6. The CPR is accessible for use in a timely way at any and all times by authorized individuals involved in direct patient care. Simultaneous and remote access to the CPR is possible.

7. The CPR system allows selective retrieval and formatting of information by users. It can present custom-tailored "views" of the same information.

8. The CPR system can be linked to both local and remote knowledge, literature, bibliographic, or administrative databases and systems (including those containing clinical practice guidelines or clinical decision support capabilities) so that such information is readily available to assist practitioners in decision making.

9. The CPR can assist and, in some instances, guide the process of clinical problem solving by providing clinicians with decision analysis tools, clinical reminders, prognostic risk assessment, and other clinical aids.

10. The CPR supports structured data collection and stores information using a defined vocabulary. It adequately supports direct data entry by practitioners.

11. The CPR can help individual practitioners and health care provider institutions manage and evaluate the quality and costs of care.

12. The CPR is sufficiently flexible and expandable to support not only today's basic information needs but also the evolving needs of each clinical specialty and subspecialty.

The committee believes that the CPR can be well established within a decade in the majority of offices of physicians, dentists, and other health care professionals and in clinics, hospitals, and multifacility provider institutions. Achieving such widespread use in only 10 years is an ambitious goal, but it can be accomplished if two conditions are met. First, a concentrated effort—with appropriate leadership, resources, coordination, and incentives—must be mounted. Second, CPR systems must be affordable and at least minimally acceptable to users.

The committee considers it essential to maintain and exploit the interest in CPRs that has been building over the past several years. A less aggressive target (e.g., 20 years) for implementation of CPRs as standard patient records could result in a loss of momentum. In contrast, a well-coordinated effort could help to accelerate progress and secure CPR implementation within the 10-year target set by the committee. The committee's remaining recommendations outline how such a concentrated effort might be organized and identify specific strategies for addressing CPR system affordability and acceptability to users.

RECOMMENDATION 2. To accomplish Recommendation 1, the committee recommends that the public and private sectors join in establishing a Computer-based Patient Record Institute (CPRI) to promote and facilitate development, implementation, and dissemination of the CPR.

The committee identified a series of activities to facilitate CPR development and implementation: (1) identification and understanding of CPR design requirements; (2) standards development; (3) research and development of CPRs and CPR systems (including networking infrastructure); (4) demonstrations of effectiveness, costs, and benefits of CPR systems; (5) review of legal constraints and needed legal protection; (6) coordination of information and resources for CPR development and diffusion; (7) coordination of information and resources for databases of secondary records; and (8) education and training of developers and users.

Some of these activities are already under way, but they are fragmented and hampered by inadequate resources and coordination. The committee believes that securing adequate resources and managing them effectively are essential to development and widespread implementation of CPR systems. To facilitate these tasks, some portion of the research devoted to CPRs should focus on the value of CPR systems. These efforts could provide potential funders of future research and development and purchasers of systems with credible evidence on which to base CPR investment decisions. Both funding and evaluation expertise from the public and private sectors should be channeled into a coordinated effort to amass this evidence. In addition, priorities should be established so that resources can be directed toward activities that promise the greatest contribution to development of CPRs and CPR systems.

Many organizations and individuals could play a role in advancing CPRs and CPR systems, but these actors are dispersed throughout the health care field and have different kinds and levels of interest in CPR development. There is no one focal point for CPR efforts and no spokesperson or organization to speak for CPR interests. Further, the nation at present has no means of developing consensus on CPR-related issues or of setting priorities among alternative uses of CPR development resources.

No existing organization has the mandate or resources for ongoing coordination of CPR resources and activities. Consequently, the committee recommends either the creation of a new organization or the extension of an existing organization's charter to achieve such coordination. For the purposes of this report, the committee has called this new or expanded component of an existing organization the Computer-based Patient Record Institute (CPRI).[1]

The CPRI has a four-part mission:

• Support the effective, efficient use of computer-based patient information in patient care, health care policymaking, clinical research, health care financing, and continuous quality improvement.

• Educate change agents and stakeholders (including the general public and health care professionals) about the value of computer-based patient records in improving patient care.

• Foster the CPR as the primary vehicle for collecting patient data.

• Promote the development and use of standards for CPR security and data content, structures, and vocabulary.

The CPRI should take several specific steps to achieve this mission:

• Establish a forum for CPR users and developers to address such issues as definition of CPR functions and content.

• Facilitate data and security standards setting and endorse such standards.

• Promote CPR data transmission through national high-speed networks by representing the biomedical community in planning for such networks.

• Address legal issues related to CPRs and CPR systems.

• Develop mechanisms for sharing the costs of acquiring and operating CPR systems among all users of CPR data.

• Define priorities and criteria for CPR demonstration projects that could be used by federal agencies, private foundations, and health care provider institutions.

• Conduct workshops and conferences to educate health care professionals and policymakers.

• Explore the need for a clearinghouse for secondary CPR information.

One of the first tasks of the CPRI should be to develop a detailed plan for achieving CPRs in terms of incremental steps that can be completed by the many individuals and organizations interested in CPR development. Such

---

[1]The name Computer-based Patient Record Institute is descriptive and not intended to limit the concept of the organization or its potential responsibility for related infrastructural issues (such as a national biomedical communications network).

a plan would establish priorities for CPR development within and among activities (e.g., define where data standards are most needed or where they could be applied most quickly). By defining and coordinating the roles of key change agents, the CPR can help focus attention on the most important tasks and avoid redundancy of effort. Moreover, by tracking and reporting concrete progress toward CPR development, the CPRI can help maintain and perhaps continue to increase interest in and resources for CPR development. It is essential that the CPRI and all organizations and individuals associated with CPR development build on existing efforts. For example, CPRI can work with the Agency for Health Care Policy and Research (AHCPR) to identify needed progress for existing databases so that secondary user needs can be better met during the transition to CPRs.

The committee, for several reasons, concluded that in the long run an independent public-private organization would be the optimal structure for the CPRI. No one federal agency would have the prestige, funding, or personnel to pursue a complete CPR agenda successfully; in addition, suspicion or skepticism on the part of the private sector (both the business and the health care communities) regarding a purely governmental effort would be difficult to overcome. The committee emphasizes that if the CPRI is to be successful, it must represent all patient record users, particularly practitioners.

A purely private sector effort also has little likelihood of success: past history shows that private sector CPR development has been fragmented, unique to particular institutions, and generally underfunded. Indeed, the base of funding in the private sector is not sufficiently solid to support a new organization at this time. In addition, it is unlikely that private sector activities can overcome intentional and unintentional governmental barriers, such as the myriad state laws and regulations that hamper progress in this area. Furthermore, certain government agencies (notably the Departments of Defense and Veterans Affairs) have made more progress in this area than the private sector, and that work should be incorporated into any national effort.

Ultimately, the committee concluded that a federally initiated and funded approach would be most appropriate for inaugurating the necessary activities. The goal of such an interim effort would be to turn over, within five years, CPR coordination efforts to a public-private organization supported by its members. The committee thus recommends a two-phase strategy for the establishment of the CPRI. In the first phase, the secretary of the Department of Health and Human Services should establish an office or program to organize specific activities aimed at reducing the barriers to computer-based patient record development. In the second phase, the CPRI should be established as a public-private organization dedicated to coordinating the many activities needed to facilitate widespread use of the CPR.

The main goals of the initial federal program should be to respond to immediate needs to advance CPR efforts and to lay the groundwork for the

CPRI. In particular, because many of the barriers to implementation relate to lack of information, the interim effort should emphasize education and evaluation of the value of CPR systems. This effort should also focus on coordinating standards development and representing the health care field's interests in the emerging national high-speed computer network.

Ideally, the interim office should be run by a small professional staff headed by a recognized expert in CPR development. An advisory board with representation from both the private and public sectors should also be established. Program staff would support standards activities, conduct educational programs, serve as liaisons to professional organizations and commissions, represent the health care community in National Science Foundation network discussions, advise AHCPR and other extramural funders of research and demonstration projects, and plan for the second phase of CPR development and implementation.

This program should be funded initially by the DHHS agencies that have a fundamental interest in patient data; these include AHCPR and other Public Health Service agencies such as the Food and Drug Administration (FDA), the Centers for Disease Control (CDC), the Health Resources and Services Administration (HRSA), and the Health Care Financing Administration (HCFA). Approximately $2 million to $5 million per year would be required for the first two years; more substantial funding would be needed for the next three years. The program should be closely aligned with AHCPR, but consideration should be given to contracting with a private sector organization to run the program. (Private sector management would allow greater flexibility and facilitate the eventual anticipated transition to a public-private entity.)

The committee urges that the private sector actively support immediate CPR activities through participation and funding (e.g., of demonstration projects) and that it be prepared to support the CPRI financially within five years. Failure of the private sector to support CPR efforts adequately could result in federal government control or dominance of CPR development and implementation efforts.

RECOMMENDATION 3. Both the public and private sectors should expand support for the CPR and CPR system implementation through research, development, and demonstration projects. Specifically, the committee recommends that Congress authorize and appropriate funds to implement the research and development agenda outlined below. The committee further recommends that private foundations and vendors fund programs to support and facilitate this research and development agenda.

Over the past several decades, impressive technological innovations in computer-based information storage, retrieval, and communication have allowed U.S. industry and research organizations to revolutionize the management of information throughout society. Yet in terms of the rapidly expanding information needs of health care, the public and private sectors have mounted only relatively limited, fragmented efforts to take advantage of these technological innovations. Most computer systems in the health care sector have evolved either from automated systems in single departments (such as the laboratory or pharmacy) or from administrative systems that support patient registration, scheduling, or financial needs. Although such systems must share data with a CPR, they cannot be used as the beginning point for its development. Major tasks in system design, computer programming, and technical integration must be completed before current technology can be exploited to speed development of the CPR. In addition, much must be learned about how the CPR can be integrated and effectively used by different health care professionals and organizations to meet their needs.

The committee strongly urges that a major research and development (R&D) effort be supported and that several demonstration prototypes of the CPR be developed, implemented, and evaluated in a variety of health care environments. Specifically, major long-term financial and organizational support for R&D and for prototype demonstration projects in implementing the CPR is greatly needed in at least six major areas: (1) data acquisition, (2) data and security standards, (3) networking support, (4) cost-benefit analysis of CPR systems, (5) CPR and quality assurance, and (6) structure and format of the patient record.

Data Acquisition

The single greatest challenge in implementing the CPR is to develop a technology that is sufficiently powerful and appropriate to the needs and preferences of health care professionals so that they can—and will—enter medical and other health care data directly into the computer. Significant new technologies (e.g., graphical user interface, voice-recognition technology, high-resolution computer displays, high-speed communication networks, and hand-held data-entry devices) can now support data entry by practitioners. These technologies hold great promise for CPR systems that will be acceptable for direct professional use. Much work, however, remains to be done to translate the potential benefits of these technologies into functioning CPR systems.

Data and Security Standards

Data Standards

Three kinds of standards apply to health data: content, data-exchange, and vocabulary. Nationally accepted standards for CPR data are of prime importance to the CPR: they are necessary for transmitting complete or partial patient records, and they are essential to the aggregation of information from many sources, either for longitudinal records of individual patients or for databases of secondary records to be used for research or epidemiological purposes. Significant efforts are under way to support standards development for CPR data dictionaries, uniform coding, vocabulary, and data formatting. More needs to be accomplished, however, before the CPR can be shared across institutions or even by different clinical information systems within institutions.

CONTENT STANDARDS Two main kinds of standards must be developed for the content of CPRs. The first requirement is a minimum data set that applies to all CPRs; the second is content standards for specific kinds of CPR records (e.g., hospital, dentist office). The lack of either of these kinds of standards will impede effective use of CPR data by clinical and nonclinical users because record content will continue to vary among practitioners and provider institutions. A further requirement is to establish a specific meaning for data elements; that is, data elements should be used to collect the same piece of information in all record systems. Efforts by various federal agencies (e.g., HCFA, DoD, VA) and health data standards groups to develop clinical data dictionaries should be coordinated to ensure a reasonable level of consistency and compatibility. The committee suggests that the CPRI foster efforts to establish a composite clinical data dictionary that would enable users to translate data from different systems to equivalent meanings.

DATA-EXCHANGE STANDARDS It is likely that patient record data will continue to be diverse because they are produced using a variety of technologies from different vendors and by a complex mix of institutions, service bureaus, reimbursement agencies, and government agencies. A major priority should be to develop and promote standards for data representation and data exchange. Without such standards, it will be impossible to support the necessary exchange of patient medical, financial, and administrative information among the different interested organizations and institutions.

In 1991, no nationally or internationally recognized format standard exists for transferring a complete patient record between disparate clinical information systems. At present, only one health data format standard (Medix, from the Institute of Electronic and Electrical Engineers) even has the objective of transferring the entire patient record, and it is not yet operational. Therefore, the CPRI should coordinate efforts to develop, test, and demonstrate a health data format standard capable of transmitting all or any portion of the CPR between different clinical systems. The committee urges that special care be taken to include input from and coordination with international standards efforts (especially those in Europe) to ensure that the format standard complies with the International Standards Organization's Open Systems Interconnect.

CLINICAL VOCABULARY STANDARDS   Effective retrieval and use of health care information in the CPR depend in large part on the consistency with which a CPR content names and describes clinical findings, clinical problems, procedures, and treatments. The development and widespread dissemination of the content and techniques of effective vocabulary control of high-priority data elements are major intellectual, technical, and organizational challenges.

Standardized vocabulary efforts such as the Unified Medical Language System (UMLS) of the National Library of Medicine (NLM) are needed to establish a common vocabulary base for clinical systems. The committee believes that funding for development of standards for clinical vocabulary systems should be expanded and, because of the technical difficulties involved, sustained for at least a decade. The committee urges that the NLM be granted increased funding over the same period to refine the UMLS further, particularly the vocabulary involved in patient care and access to clinical knowledge bases. The NLM is the appropriate organization to educate the health care community concerning UMLS and other clinical vocabulary activities, and it is well positioned to do so effectively. The CPRI could work closely with the NLM to ensure efficient, nonredundant efforts in this area.

Security Standards

PATIENT DATA CONFIDENTIALITY   Among the highest priorities in the coming decade will be the enhancement and application of methods to ensure the privacy and confidentiality of patient data in the CPR. Much of the technology to make the CPR more secure already exists, but for greatest effectiveness these technologies must be better deployed or embedded in CPR systems.

Today, no standards define the limits and scope of privacy and confidentiality for sensitive data in clinical information or CPR systems. Thus, the committee suggests that the CPRI coordinate development of such standards for health care, which will include minimal procedures with which systems must comply to ensure privacy and confidentiality in CPR systems. The institute should also address similar issues for computer systems containing secondary records (derived from data in the CPR) and establish standards for these systems as well. In particular, standards are needed to address the limits and procedures for removing (or scrambling) patient and provider identifiers in secondary records.

DATA AND SYSTEM SECURITY Standards are needed to ensure the integrity of the data in CPR systems. The committee suggests that the CPRI actively participate in developing such standards and that it coordinate and cooperate with the FDA and the Information Security Foundation proposed in the National Research Council's 1991 report, *Computers at Risk: Safe Computing in the Information Age* (published by the National Academy Press). Considerable attention was focused in the late 1980s on broad security measures for computer systems; now, the special requirements of the CPR need to be articulated and infused into the deliberations about these evolving industry standards. The committee therefore recommends that the CPRI coordinate efforts with organizations that are already active in establishing standards for secure systems and for the transmission of sensitive data over standard communications networks.

Networking Support

The information-intensive nature of health care mandates a strong emphasis on communication and transmission of information to many different organizations in diverse places. Electronic mail, file transfer, and image communication will become increasingly important support services, not only within a given hospital or health care institution but also across cities and states, and nationwide. Strong federal support will be critical for providing networking opportunities for health care information transfer at all organizational levels.

Current federal initiatives to develop high-performance national computer networks largely address the key relevant issues (enhanced transmission speeds, logistics of routing, standards for connectivity, and transmission protocols). The overall focus to date, however, has been on communications support for the research community; recognition of the role of such networks in supporting the clinical enterprise in general and the CPR in particular has been limited. To remedy this inadequacy, the CPRI should become an active participant in discussions by the Federal Networking Council regarding the National Research and Education Network.

Cost-Benefit Analysis

In view of the substantial direct costs of CPR development and implementation, issues of cost-effectiveness are important from both institutional and societal perspectives. It is not reasonable to imagine wholesale investment in and development of CPRs and CPR systems without some reliable sense of what will be gained, and at what cost. Given study time and staffing constraints, the committee did not systematically inquire into evidence regarding the cost-effectiveness of CPRs or conduct a cost-benefit

analysis. Nevertheless, it recognizes the significance of economic considerations and, as is appropriate for any new medical technology, calls expressly for an examination of the cost-effectiveness of various features of
the CPR before any widespread deployment occurs.

Major questions remain regarding the costs and benefits of the as yet
incomplete and untried technology of a comprehensive CPR and CPR system. Accurate estimates have been extremely difficult to obtain because
only incremental parts of the CPR system have been operational at any
one time. To obtain a more accurate picture of costs and benefits will
require major R&D efforts—for instance, extensive modeling and simulation projects or community-based demonstrations that could later be generalized beyond the community sites. An especially important step will be
for investigators to develop sound models of total costs and benefits
because it is likely that the CPR will range into areas of function and value
far beyond those of current patient records.

These R&D projects should address at least three issues related to the
benefits of CPRs and CPR systems. First, the nature and magnitude of
benefits to individual patients, practitioners, provider institutions, and society generally should be evaluated. Second, short-term versus long-term benefits must be examined. Third, monetary and nonmonetary benefits should
be estimated and compared. In addition, a methodological issue must be
addressed because researchers are unlikely to be able to determine benefits
in dollar terms with any precision. Thus, sophisticated approaches for char-
acterizing benefits must be employed, such as is done for complex technology assessments.

R&D efforts must also address at least two issues concerning the costs of
CPRs and CPR systems. First are the costs of acquisition, implementation,
and operation; included in these should be the costs of the R&D itself.
Second, short- and long-term costs must be appropriately identified. Cost
determinations will depend on calculation of direct costs, indirect costs, and
amortization of capitalized equipment.

Quality Assurance

The CPR can and should become a resource (with a capability far beyond
that of paper patient records) for the systematic evaluation of health care
practices and policies. The committee was unanimous in its view that, at
least on a trial basis, linking CPR information with health status assessment
provides an unprecedented opportunity to study the effectiveness and outcomes of health care procedures. Similarly, the CPR offers a vehicle for
dissemination of clinical practice guidelines.

Both individual practitioners and health care provider institutions can use
the CPR for their own purposes in evaluating and comparing patterns and

outcomes of care, and they can do so more efficiently than with a paper-based patient record system. In addition, those organizations whose responsibilities include the accreditation, regulation, and improvement of health care can, with appropriate safeguards, accumulate and analyze the data they need using the CPR rather than the paper record.

Quality of care has taken on greater salience in recent years, and public and private programs of quality assurance and continuous quality improvement have multiplied. Many of these rely (or intend to rely) on information residing in computer databases, including administrative or insurance claims files. At present, these kinds of databases are rather primitive foundations for reliable quality assurance efforts, and they have at best sparse information on important aspects of the processes and outcomes of care. Moreover, emerging efforts to develop uniform clinical data sets based on information in paper records are hampered by various drawbacks in using those records (e.g., long manual abstraction times).

Thus, CPRs and CPR systems offer great promise for furthering the nation's movement toward improving the quality of health care. Many questions, however, remain to be investigated. These include definition of minimum clinical data sets for different types and settings of care, development of appropriate real-time clinical reminders and alerts, and mechanisms for applying the statistical tools and methods of modern continuous quality improvement approaches. Although other public and private sector agencies and organizations will undoubtedly take primary responsibility for R&D in this area, the CPRI should be empowered to work directly with those groups to support these activities.

Structure and Format of the Patient Record

The technological capabilities of CPR systems offer new possibilities for improved design of patient record structure and format. To use these capabilities most effectively, the committee believes the relationship between the structure of patient records and the quality of patient care should be explored further. For example, specific elements of patient records that contribute to patient care outcomes need to be identified for incorporation into CPR systems.

The committee declined to endorse a particular patient record format at this time; rather, it strongly urges rigorous evaluation of the value of various attributes of different patient record structures.

RECOMMENDATION 4. The CPRI should promulgate uniform national standards for data and security to facilitate implementation of the CPR and its secondary databases.

As discussed earlier, major financial and organizational support is needed to promote the development of uniform national standards for data and security. Once agreed upon, these standards must be incorporated into the design and use of CPR systems; they must also be continually reviewed and revised to keep up with technological advances.

Mechanisms must be developed to communicate standards to the parties affected by them. For example, system developers and vendors should be notified when uniform national standards have been established so they can design systems with up-to-date features. System purchasers, for their part, must be educated about the value of these voluntary standards to ensure that they will buy systems that offer features that meet the standards. System users (e.g., clinicians) who may be one step removed from purchase decisions also need to be educated about standards so they can demand such features in the systems that are acquired by their institutions. Furthermore, institutions should adopt and enforce organizational policies and procedures that support standard security practices. The CPRI is an appropriate body to develop mechanisms for endorsing and communicating health care standards to affected parties.

RECOMMENDATION 5. The CPRI should review federal and state laws and regulations for the purpose of proposing and promulgating model legislation and regulations to facilitate implementation and dissemination of the CPR and its secondary databases and to streamline the CPR and CPR systems.

The committee identified at least four ways in which legal issues affect CPR development and use. First, the inconsistency of licensure laws—for instance, for hospitals across the states—can impede development and diffusion of new systems. Second, regulations can force inefficiencies on record keeping (e.g., redundant collection of data). Third, laws concerning ownership, responsibility, and control of patient records and data may be ambiguous or inconsistent, or both, and thus hinder the electronic transfer of CPR data. Fourth, laws protecting confidentiality of computer-based patient data need to be strengthened to address concerns about patient privacy.

The committee concluded that a comprehensive review of pertinent laws and regulations, especially *state* laws and regulations, is needed to remove potential legal barriers and to ensure adequate protection of patient privacy. Following this review, guidelines should be developed and disseminated to appropriate audiences. The committee noted that the Uniform Health-Care Information Act should be included in this review and that efforts should focus on why it has not been widely adopted. The committee also determined that the review process should include an assessment of and recommendations regarding penalties for violation of the privacy of patients or providers through unauthorized access or misuse of patient data in the CPR or other patient records.

The committee assigns high priority to these legal and regulatory issues because they pose major obstacles for steady progress toward the CPR and may take a long time to resolve. For this reason, the committee suggests that the CPRI convene a panel of experts to conduct such a review and prepare a report, including guidelines for state and congressional consideration. The committee also suggests that the CPRI disseminate the findings of the report through educational conferences and other means.

RECOMMENDATION 6. The costs of CPR systems should be shared by those who benefit from them. Specifically, the full costs of implementing and operating CPRs and CPR systems should be factored into reimbursement levels or payment schedules of both public and private sector third-party payers. In addition, users of secondary databases should support the costs of creating such databases.

The committee believes that capturing complete and accurate clinical data is an essential element of the patient care process; it sees the CPR as an essential tool for improving and evaluating the quality of patient care and for decreasing its costs. Short-run benefits of CPRs and CPR systems should include (1) improved patient care resulting from increased availability of patient data, medical knowledge, and clinical aids (e.g., decision support); (2) increased productivity of health care professionals from improved access to patient data and reduction of redundant data recording; and (3) reduction in administrative costs. Long-run benefits should include the ability to increase and improve medical knowledge through research using patient data derived from CPR systems.

As discussed in Chapter 4, the current distribution of costs and benefits of CPR systems may not provide adequate investment incentives for health care provider institutions. To overcome this problem, the committee believes that a better understanding of the costs and benefits of CPR systems (as discussed earlier in this chapter) and some sharing of CPR costs will be needed. Cost sharing would encourage health providers to invest in CPR systems and thus move the nation toward an optimal level of CPR system use. Further, the existence of cost-sharing mechanisms would send a signal to CPR developers regarding the strength of the CPR market and should increase the willingness of developers to invest in additional R&D.

The costs associated with CPR systems go beyond one-time procurement expenses, entailing expenditures for installation, training, maintenance, and other activities that must be planned for and appropriately budgeted. The committee therefore suggests that reimbursement mechanisms address three kinds of CPR system costs for all health care providers: (1) costs associated with procurement or leasing, (2) costs associated with installation and implementation (including training), and (3) costs associated with operation and maintenance.

The CPRI should take the lead in coordinating efforts to develop and implement reimbursement mechanisms that incorporate the costs of CPR systems. This process, which will require collaboration with representatives of practitioners, health care provider institutions, business, third-party payers, Congress, and federal and state government agencies (especially HCFA), could explore several CPR reimbursement mechanisms: incentives for data that are provided in electronic form, enhanced capital pass-through for CPR system acquisition, recognition of the costs of CPR operation in reimbursement rates, or a combination of the above. The committee urges organizations concerned with developing reimbursement levels or schedules (e.g., the Health Insurance Association of America, the Physician Payment Review Commission, the Prospective Payment Assessment Commission, and individual third-party payers) to make the establishment of acceptable CPR reimbursement mechanisms a high priority in the early 1990s.

CPR systems will greatly facilitate the creation of secondary databases for claims payment, health care policy, and clinical research by eliminating the need for manual data abstraction from records. In some cases, these databases can be constructed at a cost lower than that associated with current patient record systems; in other cases, desirable databases simply would not have been possible with current record systems. (The ability to select, retrieve, and aggregate desired data from CPRs will be of particular benefit to researchers.) Thus, users of such secondary databases should support the costs of data capture, processing, storage, and retrieval by CPR systems. The CPRI should develop an equitable plan to divide some of the costs of CPR systems that contribute to secondary databases among all such database users.

RECOMMENDATION 7. The committee recommends that health care professional schools and organizations enhance their educational programs for students and practitioners in the use of computers, CPRs, and CPR systems for patient care, education, and research.

An essential requirement for optimal functioning of CPR systems is efficient user operation of computers, CPRs, and CPR systems, including associated decision support, bibliographic retrieval, and other clinical aids. Because students and practitioners alike have educational needs in these areas, health care professional schools, programs, societies, and organizations all have a role to play in CPR education.

Such training will require curriculum modification, development of continuing postgraduate education programs, and preparation of faculty. In addition to formal training, professional schools, programs, societies, and organizations can reinforce computer skills by using computers to conduct routine business. (For example, professional societies could administer licensing examinations by computer.) The CPRI should facilitate this evolution of education programs by serving as a resource for curriculum and continuing education development.

The number of health care professionals who can design, develop, support, and train others in the use of state-of-the-art CPR systems is far fewer than the number needed. Therefore, the committee suggests that the CPRI support training programs in health care to address these personnel shortages.

The committee notes the special training needs of registered record administrators (RRAs) with respect to CPRs. As the CPR becomes more commonplace, the role of RRAs should evolve to keep pace with the changes in patient records. The RRA of the future is likely to require greater knowledge of computing technologies (including database systems and software), quality control procedures, and the needs of all patient record users. Future RRA roles may also emphasize maintaining the quality and consistency of CPRs to support patient care and facilitate research using patient data.

SUMMARY

The Institute of Medicine study committee set out to develop a plan for improving computer-based patient records and the systems in which they reside. As its first step, the committee examined why previous attempts had not resulted in wide acceptance of CPRs and asked if and how another effort might be successful. It identified five conditions in the current health care environment that it believes increase the likelihood of success: (1) ever-increasing uses of and legitimate demands for patient data, (2) availability of more powerful and more affordable technologies to support CPRs and CPR systems, (3) widespread acceptance of computers as a tool to increase efficiency in virtually all facets of everyday life, (4) an aging, mobile population, and (5) a widely held belief that needed reform in health care will not be easily achieved without routine use of CPRs.

To accomplish its task, the committee identified both the strengths and weaknesses of current patient record systems, detailed the users and uses of patient records, and defined user requirements for patient records and patient record systems. It reviewed available and emerging technologies and highlighted crucial emerging technologies whose development should be encouraged. Further, it identified nontechnological barriers to the development and diffusion of CPRs.

The committee believes its recommendations effectively address these potential barriers to routine CPR use. The first recommendation defines the CPR as the standard for future patient records. The second proposes an organizational framework within which CPR barriers can be systematically addressed and overcome. The committee's remaining recommendations then focus on specific barriers: needed research and development, promulgation of standards for CPR data and security, review of legal constraints and remedies, distribution of costs for CPR systems, and education of health care professionals.

The committee recognizes that considerable work must be accomplished and practical difficulties resolved before CPRs become the standard mode of documenting and communicating patient information and before they are perceived and used as a vital resource for improving patient care. The challenge of coordinating CPR development efforts in the pluralistic health care environment is great. Resources are limited and must be used wisely. Further, achieving maximum benefit from CPR systems will require that they be linked to an information infrastructure (i.e., network) that allows patient data, medical knowledge, and other information to be transmitted and accessed when and where needed, subject to appropriate security and confidentiality measures.

The committee is convinced that with proper coordination and appropriate resources the goal of widespread CPR utilization within a decade can be achieved. The desire to improve the quality of and access to patient data is shared by patients, practitioners, administrators, third-party payers, researchers, and policymakers across the nation. CPRs and CPR systems can respond effectively to the health care system's need for a "central nervous system" to manage the complexities of modern medicine. The CPR, in short, is an essential technology for health care.

Appendix A
Subcommittees

USERS AND USES SUBCOMMITTEE MEMBERS

Donald M. Berwick,* *Chair*, Harvard Medical School and Harvard School of Public Health, Boston, Massachusetts

Carmi Margolis, *Assistant Chair*, Ben Gurion University of the Negev, Beer-Sheva, Israel

G. Octo Barnett,* Massachusetts General Hospital, Boston

William H. Buckley, Massachusetts General Hospital, Boston

Harold D. Cross, Practitioner of Internal Medicine, Hampden, Maine

Allyson Ross Davies, New England Medical Center Hospitals, Boston, Massachusetts

Nicholas E. Davies,* Practitioner of Internal Medicine, Atlanta, Georgia

David H. Gustafson, University of Wisconsin, Madison

Clement J. McDonald, Regenstrief Institute for Health Care, Indianapolis, Indiana

Mary L. McHugh, St. Francis Regional Medical Center, Wichita, Kansas

John A. Norris,* Hill and Knowlton, Inc., Waltham, Massachusetts, and Harvard School of Public Health, Boston, Massachusetts

James S. Roberts, Joint Commission for Accreditation of Healthcare Organizations, Oakbrook Terrace, Illinois

Stephen Schoenbaum, Harvard Community Health Plan, Brookline, Massachusetts

Cary Sennett, AETNA Life Insurance Company, Hartford, Connecticut

Barclay M. Shepard, Department of Veterans Affairs, Washington, D.C.

Elaine Ullian, Faulkner Hospital, Boston, Massachusetts

Mary Joan Wogan, American Medical Record Association, Washington, D.C.

---

*Member, Committee on Improving the Patient Record.

TECHNOLOGY SUBCOMMITTEE MEMBERS

Morris F. Collen,* *Chair*, Kaiser Permanente Medical Care Program, Oakland, California

Marion J. Ball,* *Assistant Chair*, University of Maryland at Baltimore

G. Octo Barnett,* Massachusetts General Hospital, Boston

Robert J. Beck, Oregon Health Sciences University, Portland

Paul D. Clayton, Columbia Presbyterian Medical Center, New York, New York

Jerome R. Cox, Washington University, St. Louis, Missouri

Betsy L. Humphreys, National Library of Medicine, Bethesda, Maryland

Allan H. Levy, University of Illinois Medical Center, Urbana

Gretchen Murphy, Group Health Cooperative of Puget Sound, Seattle, Washington

John A. Norris,* Hill and Knowlton, Inc., Waltham, Massachusetts, and Harvard School of Public Health, Boston, Massachusetts

Helmuth F. Orthner, George Washington University, Washington, D.C.

Allan T. Pryor, University of Utah, Salt Lake City

William W. Stead, Duke University Medical Center, Durham, North Carolina

---

*Member, Committee on Improving the Patient Record.

STRATEGY AND IMPLEMENTATION SUBCOMMITTEE

Edward H. Shortliffe,* *Chair*, Stanford University School of Medicine,
  Palo Alto, California
Paul C. Tang, *Assistant Chair*, Hewlett-Packard Laboratories, Palo Alto,
  California
Margret Amatayakul, American Medical Record Association, Chicago,
  Illinois
Jeffrey F. Blair, International Business Machines Corporation, Atlanta,
  Georgia
Peter A. Bouxsein, American College of Physicians, Philadelphia,
  Pennsylvania
Nicholas E. Davies,* Practitioner of Internal Medicine, Atlanta, Georgia
Paul M. Ellwood, Interstudy, Excelsior, Minnesota
J. Michael Fitzmaurice, Agency for Health Care Policy and Research,
  Rockville, Maryland
Ruth E. Garry,* CNA Insurance Companies, Chicago, Illinois
Stephen F. Jencks, Health Care Financing Administration, Baltimore,
  Maryland
Charles N. Kahn III, U.S. House of Representatives, Committee on Ways
  and Means, Washington, D.C.
Bruce McPherson, American Hospital Association, Chicago, Illinois
Thomas Q. Morris,* Columbia Presbyterian Hospital, New York,
  New York
Jeremy Nobel, Harvard School of Public Health, Boston, Massachusetts
John A. Norris,* Hill and Knowlton, Inc., Waltham, Massachusetts, and
  Harvard School of Public Health, Boston, Massachusetts
Barclay M. Shepard, Department of Veterans Affairs, Washington, D.C.

---

*Member, Committee on Improving the Patient Record.

Appendix B

Legal Aspects of Computer-based Patient Records and Record Systems

Adele A. Waller

Computer-based patient records and record systems may bring into play laws of many kinds. For example, system hardware may be patented and system software copyrighted. If a computer-based patient record system fails and the failure results in harm to a patient, tort liability can result to the vendor or to the provider using the system, or to both. Tort liability can also arise if a system is not protected from unauthorized access and breaches of patient confidence result or records are destroyed or altered. A computer hacker gaining unauthorized access to a computerized patient record system faces possible criminal liability. Various privacy laws limit permitted disclosure or redisclosure of information stored in computer-based patient record systems.

Other laws must also be taken into account. Licensure laws applicable to health care providers, as well as reimbursement and insurance laws, all impinge on computer-based patient records, as do public health laws that require reporting of vital statistics and of various injuries and diseases. Contract law and the Uniform Commercial Code come into play in contracts for computer-based record systems. The availability of specific performance as a remedy for a vendor's breach of contract is a question that

The author is an attorney in the Health Law Department of the law firm of Gardner, Carton & Douglas, in Chicago. She gratefully acknowledges the assistance of her colleagues Deborah K. Fulton and Bernadette M. Broccolo with the computer science and computer law aspects of this paper.

200

requires resort to doctrines of equitable remedies. A hardware or software vendor's insolvency raises issues under federal bankruptcy law. Finally, interaction of computer-based record systems with artificial intelligence systems can also raise issues concerning medical device laws and, to the extent that nonphysicians are able to diagnose and treat patients without physician involvement using these systems, physician licensure laws.

Because of the plethora of laws that apply to computer-based patient records and record systems, one paper cannot encompass a full discussion of the application of these laws to the computer-based record. What follows, therefore, is a summary discussion of the key legal issues raised by computer-based patient records and record systems: regulatory and accreditation issues, evidentiary issues, patient privacy and record access concerns, record ownership questions, legal risks specific to computer-based patient record systems, and computer contracting issues.

STATE LICENSURE LAWS

Computer-based patient records utilized by an institutional health care provider must meet the requirements of relevant state licensure laws, or the institution may face licensure sanctions. The statutes and regulations governing licensure of hospitals, nursing homes, health maintenance organizations, ambulatory surgical treatment centers, and other institutional providers generally contain specific standards and requirements concerning the creation, authentication, retention, and storage of patient records, as well as limitations on the media permissible for their creation and storage. Additional requirements typically found in state licensure statutes and regulations relate to confidentiality, record content, accuracy, completeness, timeliness, and accessibility.

Hospital Licensure Laws as Barriers to Full Automation

State hospital licensure laws still pose barriers to full automation of the patient record. State-to-state variances in medical records requirements and obsolete and ambiguous or conflicting laws and regulations pose obstacles to the full development of computer-based patient record systems.[1] Although some state regulators may permit computerization of patient records in ways that technically are not permitted by state regulations, a health care institution

---

[1]State licensure requirements have lagged far behind the development of technology and have been criticized for so lagging for 20 years or more. See, e.g., Eric W. Springer, *Automated Medical Records and the Law* (Pittsburgh, Pa.: Health Law Center, 1971).

investing in an automated patient data system is making too big an investment to risk learning later that the system does not meet state licensure requirements.

Some states expressly permit use of computers in the creation, authentication, and retention of patient records.[2] Others state their medical records requirements for hospitals generally, impliedly permitting computer-based patient records, or explicitly address use of computers only for one function, such as authentication, but not for other patient record functions.[3]

Even so, the wide variance from state to state in hospital licensure requirements for medical records may make it difficult to develop patient record systems that comply with hospital licensure laws in all 50 states. State-to-state variances make it expensive to determine if a record system (or set of system specifications) complies with hospital licensure requirements in all states. They also leave open the possibility that inconsistencies between the requirements of two or more states could make it impossible for a system to meet all states' licensure requirements.

Failure by a vendor to establish a patient record system's compliance with one (or more) state's licensure requirements may adversely affect the system's marketability in such states. Assuming that hospitals include compliance with legal requirements in their feasibility analysis of computer-based patient information systems, the lack of national uniformity in the medical records requirements of state licensure laws and regulations applicable to institutional health care providers may be expected to retard development and marketing of new computer-based patient record systems. In addition, state-to-state variations in requirements regarding the content of hospital medical records may make it difficult to develop standard formats for computer-based patient records that can be used nationally.

Hospital licensure laws and regulations in many states still assume a paper patient record and at best leave the legal status of computer-based

---

[2]410 Ind. Admin. Code §15-1-9(1) (1988); Mo. Code of State Regulations, 19 C.S.R.§30-20-.021(3)(D) (1990); Oreg. Admin. Rule §333-505-050 (1989); Neb. Regulations and Standards for Hospitals §003.04 (1979); Pa. Rules and Regulations for Hospitals §115.25 (1987). In the regulations of these states, however, there is little reflection of any systematic examination of the special problems and challenges posed by automated patient records. Even Oregon, which of all the states has most systematically amended its regulations to be consistent with automated records systems, has done little more than adapt regulations from the era of paper records to permit automated patient records.

[3]22 Calif. Admin. Code §70751; Conn. Pub. Health Code, ch. 4, §19-13-03(d); 77 Ill. Admin. Code §250.1510 (1990); Lic. Stds. for Hospitals, N.J.A.C. 8:43G:-15.2; R.I. Rules and Regulations for Licensing of Hospitals §25.0 (1989); S.D. Admin. Rules §44:04:09:04 (1989); Tex. Hospital Licensing Stds. §1-22-1.4 (1985); Utah Admin. Code §R432-100-7.405 (1989); Rules and Regulations for the Lic. of Hospitals in Virginia §208.0 (1982); Wisc. Admin. Code, ch. HSS 124 Hospitals, §124.14 (1988).

patient records used by hospitals under a cloud.[4] Other state laws and regulations appear to permit some forms of automation but not others, or the use of automation for some but not all medical record functions.[5]

Oklahoma requires that all orders and medications be written in ink, a requirement that is incompatible with a fully automated medical record system. Oklahoma also prohibits substituting a signature stamp for the physician's signature, apparently requiring handwritten authentication of medical records, with the exception of records of diagnostic examinations, for which computer signatures are authorized.[6] South Carolina also requires orders to be "written in ink and signed," but permits use of a signature stamp with appropriate controls.[7] Iowa requires medical records to be "written" and "signed" by the attending physician.[8] North Carolina requires that records be "written" for all patients admitted to a hospital.[9] If a medical record must be signed in ink, the paper record—even if it is generated on a computer—becomes the original record, and many of the efficiencies of automated storage and retrieval of records cannot be realized. Other states restrict permissible medical record storage media to the original or microfilm.[10] Such a restriction is incompatible with storage of records on

---

[4]See, e.g., the rules of states that, as of the time research was completed for this paper, still required that clinical reports or clinical information be filed in or with the medical record or that records of both inpatient and outpatient treatment be filed in one folder: Ariz. Rules, Regulations and Standards for the Licensing and Regulation of Health Care Institutions §R9-10-221 (1982); Rules, Regulations and Min. Stds. for Hospitals in Idaho, IDAPA §16.02.1360.10.a; Regulations for the Licensure of General and Specialty Hospitals in the State of Maine, ch. XII (1972); Min. Stds. for Operation of Miss. Hospitals §1704.4 (1990); N.Mex. Regulations Governing General and Special Hospitals §700.B.4.f (1989); Lic. Rules for General Hospitals in North Dakota, N.D.A.C. §33-07-01-16.6.a (1990); Lic. Stds. for Hospitals and Related Institutions in the State of Oklahoma §13.5-A (1989); 64 W. Va. Legisl. Rules §10.3 (1987); Wisc. Admin. Code, ch. HSS 124 Hospitals, §124.14 (1988).

[5]See, e.g., Mo. Code of State Regulations, 19 C.S.R. §30-20.021(3)(D) (1990); Utah Admin. Code §R432-100-7.406 (1989); Hospital Rules and Regulations, Wash. Admin. Code. § 248-18-440 (1989).

[6]Licensure Standards for Hospitals and Related Institutions, State of Oklahoma §13.1-B(4) and 13.9-D (1989).

[7]S.C. Standards for Licensing Hospitals and Institutional General Infirmaries §601.6 (1990).

[8]Iowa Admin. Code §641.51.5 (1988).

[9]Rules and Statutes Applying to the Licensing of Hospitals in North Carolina, Subchapter 3c, §.1400 (1988). See also 77 Ill. Admin. Code § 250.350(a), which requires that all orders for medication and treatment be written except in emergencies. On the basis of this requirement, the Illinois Department of Public Health strongly discourages fully computerized medical records in hospitals.

[10]See, e.g., Colo. General Hospitals, ch. IV, §4.2 (1982); Conn. Pub. Health Code, ch. 4, §19-13-03(d) (1989); 410 Ind. Admin. Code §15-1-9(2)(b)(1) (1988); Regulations for the Licensure

computer disks, magnetic tape, or optical disks—that is, unless the records were both originally created and authenticated by computer and are permanently retained on the original medium (which may be difficult or infeasible, depending on the medium's durability).

A serious legal barrier to full realization of the potential of computer-based patient records is the confusion and lack of clarity in some states' standards when they are applied to computer-based medical records.

It is not always clear whether regulations requiring that records be kept in ink or "type" (or in ink or "typewritten") permit creation of medical records electronically or with the use of lasers, although a provision permitting authentication of records by computer key, such as that found in Colorado's rules, implies that patient records may be created on a computer.[11] Similarly, it is unclear whether a requirement that medical records be recorded in ink, typewritten, or recorded electronically permits recording by lasers on optical disks.[12]

The regulations of some states require that medical records be "signed" but are silent on whether the substitution of a computer key or code for a physician's signature is permitted.[13] This silence cannot be interpreted as

---

of General and Specialty Hospitals in the State of Maine, ch. XII (1972); Min. Stds. for Operation of Miss. Hospitals §1702 (1990); Mo. Code of State Regulations, 19 C.S.R. §30-20.021(3)(D) (1990); Operational Rules and Regulations for Health Facilities, Nev. Admin. Code §449.379 (1988); N.Mex. Regulations Governing General and Special Hospitals §700.B.1.b (1989); S.C. Standards for Licensing Hospitals and Institutional General Infirmaries §601.6 (1990); Tenn. Hospitals Rules and Regulations §1200-8-4-.03(f) (1986); Wisc. Admin. Code, ch. HSS 124 Hospitals, §124.14 (1988). Tennessee has recently amended its statute to permit storage of medical records on "non-erasable optical and electronic imaging technology." See Tenn. Code Ann. § 68-11-306(b) (1991).

[11]See, e.g., Rules of Alabama State Bd. of Hlth., Div. of Lic. and Cert., Hospitals, §420-5-7.07(f) (1988); Rules and Regulations for Hospitals and Related Institutions in Arkansas §0601(C) (1988); Colo. General Hospitals, ch.IV, §4.4 (1982); Tenn. Hospitals Rules and Regulations §1200-8-4-.03 (1986); Vermont Lic. Stds. for the Construction, Maintenance and Operations of Hospitals §3-946 (1954); 64 W. Va. Legisl. Rules §10.3 (1987).

[12]Mo. Code of State Regulations, 19 C.S.R. §30-20.021(3)(D) (1990).

[13]See, e.g., Ariz. Rules, Regulations and Standards for the Lic. and Regulation of Health Care Institutions §R9-10-221 (1982); Conn. Pub. Health Code, ch. 4, §19-13-03(d) (1989); Ga. Rules and Regulations for Hospitals §290-5-6-.11 (1977); Rules, Regulations and Min. Stds. for Hospitals in Idaho, IDAPA §16.02.1360.13; Iowa Admin. Code §641.51.5 (1988); Ky. 902 KAR 20:016 (1989); Min. Stds. for Operation of Miss. Hospitals §1704.4 (1990); Nev. Operational Rules and Regulations for Health Facilities §449.379; N.Mex. Regulations Governing General and Special Hospitals §700; Lic. Rules for General Hospitals in North Dakota, N.D.A.C. §33-07-01-16.9 (1990); Lic. Stds. for Hospitals and Related Institutions in the State of Oklahoma §13.5-A (1989); S.C. Standards for Licensing Hospitals and Institutional General Infirmaries §601 (1990); Tenn. Hospitals Rules and Regulations §1200-8-4-.03 (1986); Vermont Lic. Stds. for the Construction, Maintenance and Operations of Hospitals §3-946 (1954); 64 W.Va. Legisl. Rules §10.3 (1987); Wisc. Admin. Code, ch. HSS 124 Hospitals, §124.14 (1988); Wy. Stds., Rules and Regulations for Hospitals and Related Facilities §7 (1979).

necessarily permitting authentication of records by computer key or code. In addition, many states require that each patient's record contain a "signed" consent form or evidence of informed consent.[14] It is not clear whether paper files of consent forms must be maintained or whether it is permissible for patients and patient representatives to authenticate consent on a computer by use of a computer key or code unique to each patient.

State requirements that medical records (or "original" medical records) be retained in the hospital or on the hospital's premises, except under defined circumstances, mean that use of outside computer services for hospital medical records may constitute a technical violation of the hospital licensure requirements in some states.[15] Indiana's regulations, although containing a provision that a computerized record shall be considered the same as a written record, also require that medical records be filed in a safe, accessible manner in the hospital and be kept on the nursing unit during the patient's hospitalization. These two requirements leave the status of outside computer services for Indiana hospitals unclear.[16]

Other State Licensure Laws

State licensure laws and regulations applicable to a variety of other health care providers—both institutional and individual—typically contain provisions concerning patient records or patient information and confidences, or both.

State laws and regulations with respect to licensure of institutional providers other than hospitals contain many of the same types of patient record requirements and raise many of the same issues raised by hospital licensure laws and regulations. Licensure laws and regulations for such providers may pose even greater barriers to fully computer-based patient records be-

---

[14]See, e.g., N.J. Lic. Stds. for Hospitals, N.J.A.C. 8:43G-15.2(d)(1) (1990).

[15]Rules and Regulations for Hospitals and Related Institutions in Arkansas §0601(V) (1988); Conn. Pub. Health Code, ch. 4, §19-13-03(d)(6) (1989); 410 Ind. Admin. Code §15-1-9(2) (1988); Iowa Admin. Code §641.51.5(1) (1988); Ky. 902 K.A.R. §20:016 (1989); Regulations for the Licensure of General and Specialty Hospitals in the State of Maine, ch. XII (1972); Min. Stds. for Operation of Miss. Hospitals §1701.4 (1990); N.J. Lic. Stds. for Hospitals, N.J.A.C. 8:43G-15.2(h) (1990); N.Mex. Regulations Governing General and Special Hospitals §700.B.1.b (1989); Rules and Statutes Applying to the Licensing of Hospitals in North Carolina, Subchapter 3c, §.1403(d) (1988); Licensure Standards for Hospitals and Related Institutions, State of Oklahoma §13.2-C (1989); Pa. Rules and Regulations for Hospitals §115.28 (1987); S.C. Standards for Licensing Hospitals and Institutional General Infirmaries §601.4 (1990); Tenn. Hospitals Rules and Regulations §1200-8-4-.03(b)(1) (1986); 64 W. Va. Legisl. Rules §10.3.1(a) (1987); Wisc. Admin. Code, ch. HSS 124 Hospitals, §124.14(2) (1988).

[16]410 Ind. Admin. Code §15-1-9 (1988).

cause, even more than hospital licensure laws and regulations, they may be keyed to a paper record.

For example, Illinois' long-term care facility licensure regulations require that (1) resident records be written in ink or typed and (2) all physician orders, plans of treatment, Medicare and Medicaid certifications and recertification statements, and similar documents have the original written signature of the physician. Use of a rubber stamp signature, with or without initials, is not permitted. In addition, resident records must contain a "physician's order sheet," a "medication sheet," and "treatment sheets," implying that a manual record must be maintained.[17]

State licensure requirements for nonhospital institutional providers exhibit the same lack of national uniformity in standards for patient records exhibited by state hospital licensure requirements. In addition, similar concerns regarding obsolete and ambiguous laws and regulations arise in state licensure requirements for institutional providers other than hospitals.

State laws and regulations applicable to physicians, nurses, and other individuals licensed to provide health care typically contain an express or implied obligation of confidentiality with respect to patient confidences and, in some statutes or regulations, with respect to patient records. Willful or negligent breaches of confidentiality may constitute grounds for professional discipline.[18]

The canons of ethics of a profession may be incorporated into a state's licensure requirements, usually by a provision in a licensing act that makes "unprofessional conduct" grounds for professional discipline.[19] The 1989 publication *Current Opinions of the Council on Ethical and Judicial Affairs of the American Medical Association* contains detailed guidelines on computerized patient databases.[20] These may be impliedly incorporated into the statutes and regulations governing licensure of physicians in some states.

Medicare Regulations

To participate in the Medicare program, a provider must meet the applicable Medicare conditions of participation. The conditions of participation for hospitals include requirements for medical records but do not include

---

[17]77 Ill. Admin. Code §300.1810 (1985).

[18]See, e.g., 111 Ill. Ann. Stat. ¶4400-22.30 (Smith-Hurd 1990 Supplementary Pamphlet).

[19]See, e.g., 52 Oreg. Rev. Stat. §677.188 (1989); Utah Code Ann. §58-12-35 (1990).

[20]American Medical Association (AMA), Chicago, Illinois. Although it may not be practical to implement all of the AMA's guidelines, it should be recognized that these guidelines are some of the most detailed, ethically sensitive standards for computerized patient databases that have been developed to date.

any express restriction on permissible media for creating and storing medical records.[21] Medical records may be authenticated by signature, written initials, or computer entry.[22] Thus, the conditions of a hospital's participation in the Medicare program pose no barrier to the use of computer-based patient records.

The Medicare conditions of participation for long-term care facilities do not expressly restrict the media for creation and storage of the records.[23] However, they require each individual who completes a portion of the assessment to "sign" the assessment.[24] In addition, these conditions of participation require that, at each visit to a resident, the physician supervising the resident's medical care must "write, sign and date progress notes" and "sign all orders."[25] It is not clear whether these conditions of participation permit a fully automated record because it is not clear whether authentication by computer code or key provides the required signature and whether a progress note made on a computer fulfills the requirement that a physician must write the note.[26]

The Health Care Financing Administration (HCFA) permits physician certifications of medical necessity to be executed by computer or transmitted to a hospital by facsimile machines. A provider seeking permission for its physicians to attest to medical necessity on a computer or by facsimile must be able to demonstrate to its intermediary that its system contains adequate safeguards of accuracy and confidentiality and meets certain other standards.[27]

---

[21]42 C.F.R. §482.24.

[22]42 C.F.R. §482.24(c)(1)(ii).

[23]42 C.F.R. §483.75(n).

[24]42 C.F.R. §483.20(c)(2).

[25]42 C.F.R. §483.40(b).

[26]Apparently, the Health Care Financing Administration (HCFA) believes that these conditions of participation would permit a fully automated record because HCFA is discussing with nursing home operators the possibility of requiring that nursing homes computerize resident assessment records to comply with the provision of the Omnibus Budget Reconciliation Act of 1987 requiring maintenance of a uniform, minimum data set on residents' conditions. See Paula Eubanks, "Homes Doubt They Can Computerize per HCFA's Request," *Hospitals* 64, no. 23 (1990):56.

[27]See the HCFA Medicare Hospital Manual Transmittal No.567 (July 1989). The provider's request must explain (1) the provider's physician identification system, (2) system safeguards to ensure confidentiality, (3) how data are displayed for physician review before electronic attestation, (4) how physician identity is determined upon certification and stored in the provider's system, (5) how the system records a system-generated date and time of entry at the point of attestation, (6) system backup procedures for prolonged downtime, and (7) how the physician verifies that attestations executed through the system have been correctly recorded. HCFA permits use of physician access systems that employ an alphanumeric identifier or biometric identification of physicians.

Hospital Accreditation Requirements

Technically, the Joint Commission on Accreditation of Healthcare Organizations (JCAHO) is a voluntary organization, and JCAHO accreditation is voluntary. JCAHO accreditation standards, however, are incorporated in some state hospital licensure laws, at least in part,[28] and a hospital is deemed to meet certain Medicare conditions of participation if it holds JCAHO accreditation.[29]

Although JCAHO accreditation standards do not explicitly address required media for record keeping and storage, they assume that a hospital may participate in an automated medical record data processing system. JCAHO standards permit authentication of medical records by computer key.

The JCAHO requires that all medical records be accurate, accessible, authenticated, organized, confidential, secure, current, legible, and complete.[30] A computer-based medical record system can meet JCAHO standards if the system is properly designed and maintained and if medical records are otherwise properly completed.

PATIENT RIGHTS ISSUES

Right of Privacy

The Federal Privacy Act and similar acts in many states provide assurance that patient records held by the federal government and governments of states that have enacted privacy legislation will not be disclosed to third parties without the patient's consent, except under defined circumstances.[31] However, privacy of patient records in other states and in the private sector is governed by a crazy quilt of statutory, regulatory, and common-law rules and is often inadequately protected.[32]

Growing demands for information contained in patient records pose an ever-increasing threat to patient privacy. Such demands come not only

---

[28]See, e.g., the following regulations, which incorporate JCAHO standards for medical records into state hospital licensure requirements: N.H. Code of Admin. Rules, Part He-P802 (1986); R.I. Rules and Regulations for Licensing of Hospitals §25.7; Rules and Regs. for the Licensure of Hospitals in Virginia §208.5 (1982).

[29]42 U.S.C. §1395bb.

[30]Joint Commission on Accreditation of Healthcare Organizations, "Medical Record Services (MR)," *Accreditation Manual for Hospitals* (Chicago: 1990).

[31]5 U.S.C. §552a.

[32]The threats to patient privacy posed by increased use of computers for health records were detailed by Alan F. Westin in *Computers, Health Records and Citizen Rights* (Washington, D.C: U.S. Government Printing Office, 1976).

from peer-review bodies, third-party payers (both governmental and non-governmental), outside billing and computer services, and government, but from employers, insurers, and others who use health care information for non-health care purposes.

When information from patient records is disclosed by a provider—whether with or without the patient's consent—it is extremely difficult to control redisclosure of the information effectively, even though confidentiality agreements and notices are still advisable. Furthermore, when patient records are computerized, they can easily be transmitted across state lines, limiting the ability of any one state to protect the privacy of its citizens.

To the extent that patients and providers are aware that computer-based patient records increase the threat to patient privacy, they may be unwilling to provide or record complete information in the patient record, particularly with regard to sensitive matters, such as abortions, AIDS (acquired immune deficiency syndrome), psychiatric problems, and drug or alcohol abuse. Thus, the lack of adequate, uniform, national protection of patient privacy with respect to patient records may hinder full development of computer-based patient record systems.

The Uniform Health-Care Information Act skillfully addresses issues of confidentiality and release of patient information.[33] Only Montana, however, has enacted this act into law.[34]

Right of Access to Health Records

Most states expressly allow a patient or a patient's authorized representative to inspect and copy the patient's hospital records.[35] Rights of access to health records maintained by physicians and other individual health care providers may not always be clear.

Before records become available, the person seeking access typically must request such access in writing from the provider and pay reasonable clerical costs. A few states grant patients the right to review their hospital records only after discharge.[36]

Many states permit providers to refuse to grant a patient's request for disclosure where psychiatric records are involved and where release of the information would be detrimental to the patient's mental health or general

---

[33]National Conference of Commissioners on Uniform State Laws, *Uniform Laws Annual*, vol. 9, part 1 (St. Paul, Minn.: West Publishing Co., 1988), p. 475.

[34]M.C.A. §50-16-501, *et seq.*

[35]See, e.g., Ala. Stat. §18.23.065.

[36]See, e.g., Fla. Stat. Ann. §395.017(1); Ill. Ann. Stat., ch. 110, §8-2001.

health, or where a third party could be endangered by the release.[37] However, in such states, a provider may be required to deliver copies of the record to the patient's representative or attorney.

Several statutes contain special provisions concerning a patient's access to particular portions of his or her record, such as X-rays.[38] Still other states allow a provider to prepare a summary of the patient's record for inspection and copying rather than allowing the patient access to the entire record.[39] In the absence of statute or regulation, some courts have recognized a provider's common-law duty to allow a patient limited access to his or her records.[40]

Where patient records become part of insurers' or other databases, the patient may not even know that the record exists and may have no way to enforce a right of access, even if such exists. In addition, even if the patient gains access to the record, he or she may have no legally enforceable right to correct inaccurate information contained in it.

The Uniform Health-Care Information Act addresses access issues, as well as issues of confidentiality and information disclosure.[41] As noted earlier, however, only Montana has adopted this legislation to date.[42] Issues of access to databases maintained by insurers, correction of data maintained on individuals by insurance companies, and limitations on redisclosure of such information are addressed in the Insurance Information and Privacy Protection Model Act developed by the National Association of Insurance Commissioners (NAIC). To date, at least 13 states have adopted some version of this model act as law.[43]

---

[37]See, e.g., Fla. Stat. Ann. §395.017(1); Okla. Stat. Ann., ch. 76, §19A; Cal. Health & Safety Code Ann. §1795.14(b); Colo. Rev. Stat. §25-1-801; Hawaii Rev. Stat. Ann. §622-57; Maine Rev. Stat. Ann. §1711; Minn. Stat. Ann. §144.335.

[38]See, e.g., Cal. Health & Safety Code Ann. §1795.12(c) and (e).

[39]See, e.g., Cal. Health & Safety Code Ann. §1795.20(a); Minn. Stat. Ann §144.335.

[40]See, e.g., *Cannell v. Medical and Surgical Clinic*, 21 Ill. App. 3d 383, 315 N.E. 2d 278 (1974); *Matter of Weiss*, 208 Misc. 1010, 147 N.Y.S. 2d 455 (N.Y. Spec. Term. 1955); *Hutchins v. Texas Rehab. Comm.*, 544 S.W. 2d 802 (Tex. Civ. Ct. App. 1976).

[41]9 Uniform Laws Ann., Part 1 (West 1988), p. 475.

[42]M.C.A. §50-16-501, *et seq.*

[43]The NAIC model act is a good beginning but does not go far enough in protecting individuals whose health records are disclosed to insurance companies. One Kansas court, for example, found that transmission of health information concerning the plaintiff to the Medical Information Bureau did not invade the plaintiff's privacy (*Senogles v. Security Benefit Life Insurance Co.*, 217 Kan. 438, 536 P. 2d 1358 [1975]). The Medical Information Bureau is a nonprofit association formed to conduct a confidential exchange of information between its more than 700 insurance company members, which pool information on underwriting decisions and the health status of individual insureds.

Ownership of Patient Data and of the Patient Record

Ownership of the Patient Record

It is generally accepted that a provider owns the physical patient records created by the provider in delivering care to patients, subject to the patient's limited interest in the information contained in the record.[44]   This rule concerning ownership of the patient record is established by statute in some states and by regulation in others (e.g., hospital licensure regulations).[45] In the absence of statutory or regulatory authority, a few courts have held that a medical record is the property of the provider, subject to the limited property interest of the patient in the information contained in the record.[46]

Rights in Information Contained in the Record

Provider ownership of patient records does not imply that the provider has a right to use, disclose, or withhold data in the record at will. Patients generally have a qualified property interest in the information contained in their medical records. However, the precise limits of this interest vary from state to state.

EVIDENTIARY ISSUES

Importance of Admissibility of Patient Records as Evidence

A computer-based patient record system should be structured so that patient records created and stored on the system can be admitted as evidence in court in disputes between providers and patients or payers, in cases in which the medical condition of the patient is at issue, and in other litigation. Because records of many businesses are computerized, courts have developed standards for establishing the trustworthiness of computerized records.

---

[44]See, e.g., *Position Statement, Confidentiality of Patient Health Information* (American Medical Record Association, 1985); Joint Commission on Accreditation of Healthcare Organizations, "MR 3.1," *Accreditation Manual for Hospitals* (Chicago: 1990).

[45]See, e.g., Tenn. Code Ann. §68-11-304; Mo. Rules of Dept. of Health, 19 C.S.R. §30-20.021(D)(6) (1990).

[46]See, e.g., *Bishop Clarkson Memorial Hospital v. Reserve Life Insurance Co.*, 350 F.2d 1006 (8th Cir. 1965); *Pyramid Life Insurance Co. v. Masonic Hospital Association of Payne County*, 191 F.Supp. 51 (W.D. Okla. 1961); *Thurman v. Crawford*, 652 S.W. 2d 240 (Mo. App. 1983); *Hutchins v. Texas Rehab. Comm.*, 544 S.W. 2d 802 (Tex. Civ. App. 1976); *Morris v. Hoerster*, 377 S.W. 2d 840 (Tex. Civ. App. 1964).

Rule Against Hearsay

Definition of Hearsay

Hearsay is generally defined as a statement out of court by a declarant offered as evidence to prove the truth of the matter asserted in the out-of-court statement.[47] Hearsay is not admissible as evidence in court unless one of the many exceptions to the hearsay rule applies.[48] All medical records, including computer-based records, are hearsay.

Business Records Exception

To come within the business record exception to the rule against hearsay, records must be kept regularly in the ordinary course of business and not be specially prepared for trial. In addition, record entries must have been made at or near the time the events recorded. The identity of the person making or recording the entries must be captured in the record; in addition, the record must have been prepared by or from information transmitted by a person with firsthand knowledge of the event recorded who is acting in his or her ordinary business capacity.[49]

A computer-based medical record made in the normal manner at the time of delivering care should meet the requirement that a business record be kept regularly in the ordinary course of business. Providers should ensure that the computer records the date and time of each entry and update to a medical record so that the time and timeliness of that entry or update can be demonstrated in court.

The computer should also record the identity of each person who makes an entry or modifies a record. Ensuring the integrity of a system's record of identity may be difficult if records are created directly on the system by health professionals—they could share or discover each other's computer passwords and key codes. A system of key cards and secret passwords similar to those used on automatic teller machines may provide greater integrity. Strict rules against disclosing passwords and codes should be publicized to all system users and should be strictly enforced. A provider may want to consider a system that verifies the identity of users by voice- or thumbprint; however, the cost of such sophisticated features may be prohibitive.

---

[47]See, e.g., Rule 801(c), Federal Rules of Evidence, and Rule 801(c), Uniform Rules of Evidence.

[48]See, e.g., Rule 802, Federal Rules of Evidence, and Rule 802, Uniform Rules of Evidence.

[49]See, e.g., Rule 803(6), Federal Rules of Evidence, and Rule 803(6), Uniform Rules of Evidence.

When an error is corrected in a computerized record, the system should preserve both the original entry and the correction, along with the identity of the person making the correction. Otherwise, it may appear that a record has been altered as part of a cover-up or that records on the system are not sufficiently reliable to be trustworthy as evidence and, thus, are not admissible in court.

Write-once, read-many (WORM), or compact disk, read-only memory (CD-ROM), technology may be attractive in this context because disks cannot be altered once information is recorded. Write-protecting the portions of computer disks on which patient information is stored can also protect the integrity of records stored on a computerized patient record system. However, reliable software that preserves erroneous entries and tracks the history of each entry and correction to a record should provide adequate demonstration of the reliability of the record to a court.

A provider should have an employee or technical consultant who can testify concerning the reliability of the system's identification and entry-dating process and the trustworthiness of the system as a whole, including system security features and procedures.

Records stored on a properly designed and maintained computer-based system should come within the business records exception to the hearsay rule if the guidelines above are followed. Statements contained in such computerized records will generally be admissible if made by providers or their staffs acting in the ordinary course of business. Statements contained in such records may also be admissible if made by the declarant "for purposes of medical diagnosis or treatment and describing medical history, or past or present symptoms, pain, or sensations, or the inception or general character of the cause or external source thereof insofar as reasonably pertinent to diagnosis or treatment."[50]

Best Evidence Rule

The evidentiary rules of some jurisdictions provide that, in instances in which the contents of a writing are at issue, the original document must be proffered unless an exception to the rule is satisfied. The Federal Rules of Evidence state that "[i]f data are stored in a computer or similar device, any printout or other output readable by sight, shown to reflect the data accurately, is an 'original.'" The federal rules also provide for admissibility of duplicates to the same extent as originals unless a genuine issue of authen-

---

[50]Rule 803(4), Federal Rules of Evidence. This exception to the hearsay rule is known as the medical records exception.

ticity or unfairness arises.[51] Some states' evidentiary rules also accept computerized documents as originals.[52]

Other states permit reproductions to be admitted as evidence when such copies are made in the regular course of business and satisfy other criteria for trustworthiness.[53] The trustworthiness of an automated system refers to the reliability of system hardware and software, the use of proper procedures for creating and storing records, the assurance that entries are made by adequately trained personnel, and the prevention of unauthorized access to the records and of tampering with the system.

RISKS ARISING FROM COMPUTER-BASED PATIENT RECORD SYSTEMS

Breaches of Confidentiality and Unauthorized Access

The duty of health care providers to maintain the confidentiality of patient records and to protect them from unauthorized access arises from licensure laws and regulations, specific statutes and regulations with respect to certain patient records (e.g., alcohol and drug abuse patient records, psychiatric records, and records of positive human immunodeficiency virus [HIV] antibody test results), JCAHO standards, Medicare rules, and the common law. In addition, the necessity of keeping records in a manner that makes them admissible as evidence in court requires a provider to protect patient records from unauthorized access.

The legal duties to preserve confidentiality and prevent unauthorized access to patient records are the same with respect to both paper and computer-based records. However, keeping computer-based records confidential and free from unauthorized access poses special challenges, and a failure to do so can have more onerous consequences than may occur in the case of paper records.

The computer's capacity for collecting, storing, and permitting access to large quantities of information often means that more information is collected and stored on computer-based record systems than is collected and stored in paper records. Because of the computer's capacity for mass storage and copying, one breach of a system's security can result in the unauthorized disclosure of extensive information about large numbers of patients. In addition, the computer's capacity to provide health information on large numbers of patients at one time makes computer-based patient

---

[51]Rules 1001(3) and 1003.
[52]See, e.g., Fla. Stat. Ann. §90.951.
[53]See, e.g., Cal. Evid. Code §§1270-1272.

record systems an even more tempting target than paper records. As the medical information included in patient records becomes more sophisticated (e.g., genetic information), this temptation will only increase.

Mass disclosure of patient information could result in catastrophic liability for a provider; it could also result in licensure sanctions or statutory penalties. Theories under which providers may be held liable for breaches of confidentiality include both statutory and common-law theories. Common-law theories under which providers may be held liable for breaches of confidentiality include invasion of privacy, betrayal of professional secrets, breach of contract, slander, and negligent or intentional infliction of emotional distress. Statutes such as the federal statute concerning confidentiality of drug and alcohol abuse patient records provide penalties for breaches.

Security mechanisms and procedures can provide some level of protection to computer-based patient records against unauthorized access by users both inside and outside a provider organization. Yet even the most sophisticated security measures will not provide fail-safe protection of patient records, particularly in decentralized systems. In fact, one of the biggest threats to the security of computer-based patient records comes from the trend toward networked systems. Security measures that are both adequate and affordable and that do not interfere with efficient patient care currently do not exist for such systems.

A computer-based patient record system should include a security system that, as far as is practicable, permits only authorized users to access patient records and permits authorized users to access only those portions of the records that are relevant to their particular functions. The system should also ensure that access to each record is tracked by the system and monitored as a deterrent to unauthorized review of records. Access to sensitive records or portions of records should be sharply limited; this kind of access should also be tracked by the system and carefully monitored by the provider. Such records include HIV-antibody test results, records of drug and alcohol abuse patients, psychiatric records, and records of celebrity patients. With AIDS patients, the main and more easily accessible portion of the record can include a notation to use body fluid precautions without identifying the patient as having AIDS, hepatitis, or some other disease transmissible by body fluids. HIV-antibody test results can either be omitted from the automated system or stored in a restricted portion of the record. To the extent that sensitive records are not stored on the system, however, the advantages of a totally automated system cannot be realized.

A provider with a computer-based patient record system that uses passwords, access codes, and key cards should have and strictly enforce policies against disclosing or sharing such means of access. Alternatively, a provider could use a system that identifies users biometrically through voiceprints, thumbprints, or other unique individual features; however, the sophisticated technology required for this kind of system may still be prohibitively expensive for many health care providers. In a hospital, policies against sharing passwords, access codes, and key cards should apply to the medical staff as well as to employees. Violation of these policies should be grounds for discipline, up to and including termination of employment or revocation of medical staff membership. When employment or medical staff membership ends, computer access should terminate immediately.

Hospital medical staff members should be asked to sign confidentiality statements acknowledging that passwords, access codes, and key cards are for personal use only. Physicians should be held liable for any entries to a record made by nurses or assistants using the physician's password.

To discourage password and access code sharing, an individual should be available 24 hours a day to assist authorized users who forget their access codes and persons with a legitimate need for one-time record access. An institution should also develop a mechanism for overriding the computer security system in the event of an emergency.

The use of computer networking, computer facilities owned or operated by others, or computer sharing could result in unauthorized access to computer-based records and breaches of confidentiality. In addition, outside computer consultants and technicians (including service personnel and vendor representatives) who obtain access to a computer-based patient record system conceivably could access records in an unauthorized manner or breach confidentiality. Thus, a provider should enter into confidentiality agreements with all outsiders who may have access to medical records and should have appropriate hardware and software security.

To protect against mass access and extraction of information from a computer-based patient record system, the system should include special security measures against programs that permit mass copying of records at one time or that have the potential to access or alter large numbers of records at one time.

Current computer security technology cannot provide perfect security for computer-based patient record systems. The security mechanisms available for decentralized systems and computer networks provide much less protection than those available for mainframe systems. Given current technology, the need for security generally must be balanced with the need of health care professionals and hospital staff for easy, immediate access to patient records.

Currently feasible security measures are particularly inadequate for networked systems and probably cannot protect providers that install computer-based record systems from substantial exposure to liability. To the extent that providers are aware of this exposure, they may be deterred from using computer-based patient record systems.

Computer Viruses and Other Computer Sabotage

Computer viruses and other forms of computer sabotage pose real threats to the integrity of computer-based patient record systems. Viruses or other forms of sabotage can result in the alteration or destruction of data or the creation of false data on the system; they can also cause the system to slow down or crash or otherwise make patient records inaccessible, either temporarily or permanently.

Sabotage can be carried out by both insiders and outsiders and by both authorized and unauthorized system users. Health care providers cannot discount the possibility of sabotage by disgruntled employees. In fact, the biggest threat to system integrity and patient record confidentiality comes from employees and other insiders.

The risk of viruses or other sabotage from the outside can be substantially reduced by eliminating all networking and electronic data sharing with outside computers and by not using any disk from an outside source. Such isolation of a system is generally infeasible, however, and would rule out hospital-physician office linkages and other networking for which there may be important clinical or research reasons. Antivirus software can aid in blocking or detecting viruses and other sabotage.

Software vendors have been known to sabotage a system when payment has been withheld for a system's failure to meet contractual standards. Therefore, a system purchaser or lessor should consider insisting that vendors indemnify the purchaser against all damage and losses resulting from keylocks, viruses, worms, bombs, and the like inserted into software by the vendor or its agents, and from other computer sabotage by the vendor or its agents.

Providers using computer-based record systems have a legal obligation to take security measures that are reasonable, at least by current standards. Currently available security technology for networked patient record systems is insufficient to give providers total assurance that the confidentiality of their records will not be breached or that the integrity of patient records on the system cannot be destroyed. One catastrophic incident involving a computer-based patient record system could set the legal status of computer-based record systems back decades. Therefore, development of improved security technology is of utmost importance.

Potential for Inaccessibility

Medicare, the JCAHO, and most state hospital licensure laws require that medical records for current hospital patients be readily accessible and stored in a way that permits prompt retrieval of information. Keeping computer-based patient records available means minimizing system downtime and having adequate backup mechanisms.

In addition to its potential for hindering patient care, which may result in negligence liability, excessive patient record system downtime may also create regulatory violations or JCAHO accreditation deficiencies. The following precautions can help protect against inaccessibility of computer-based patient records:

1. properly maintaining hardware and thoroughly debugging and maintaining system software;
2. ascertaining other users' experience with system downtime and their ability to bring a system back up quickly prior to contracting for purchase or lease of a system;
3. including performance standards in any lease or contract with a vendor, as well as guarantees of reliability and of ongoing maintenance support;
4. taking adequate precautions against sabotage of the system; and
5. having adequate backup and emergency capability.

Questions of Durability

Medical records must be durable for a number of reasons: to meet state licensure requirements, to comply with Medicare rules, to preserve a record of patient encounters for use as evidence in malpractice and other lawsuits, to permit future treatment of the patient or future notification to patients who have received treatment that creates health risks for them or their descendants, and, in some cases, to support research. Some states require hospitals to retain medical records for 25 years.[54] A researcher or research institution may need to preserve medical records for as long as 75 years.

Changes in technology that cause patient record systems to become obsolete before the need for records stored on the systems has ended can mean that old and new systems do not interface. Another potential risk is that unproven new technology may lack durability. For example, the long-term durability of optical disks has not yet been proven.

Copying patient records from an old system to a new system raises special concerns. Reliable evidence of the chain of copying must be preserved so that the copied records can be admitted as evidence in court. The provider must also ensure that copied records comply with a state's hospital and other institutional licensure requirements as to the media in which patient records can be retained.

---

[54]Conn. Public Health Code §19-13-D3(e)(6); Nev. Operational Rules and Regulations for Health Facilities §449.379-2 (1988); Lic. Rules for General Hospitals in N. Dakota §33-07-01-16.3 (1990).

Accuracy Issues

Errors in computer-based patient records can result from faulty software or equipment or from human error. A patient record system should be free from significant errors in computer hardware and software. Laboratory equipment and other machines providing input to a computer-based patient record system should also be free from such errors.

Mechanisms for minimizing human error, such as reviews of input for accuracy, are also advisable. When corrections are made, they should be logged on the system as suggested in the previous section concerning evidentiary issues. If clinical observations are recorded using bar coding or other programmed codes, there should be a mechanism in place for visual confirmation or other verification of the codes entered into the computer.

Selected Legal Issues in Computer Contracting

Leases and acquisitions of computers may involve some or all of the following: hardware, operating, and application software licenses; installation, testing, and implementation services; and postinstallation maintenance and support services for both operating and application software and equipment. Use of multiple agreements to address these interrelated components of computer system acquisitions creates the risk of conflict among the agreements and may confuse even more the issues of what law applies to these agreements. Unless multiple agreements cannot be avoided (e.g., different vendors for the hardware/operating software and application software), a single agreement is preferable.

Because of the hybrid nature of contracts for computer systems, it is not always clear what law governs issues of contract interpretation, the rights of the parties, procedures for resolving disputes, and so forth. If a court characterizes a transaction as a sale of goods, the Uniform Commercial Code will apply. However, computer system acquisitions involve both goods and services and often involve licenses rather than sales of software (to which the Uniform Commercial Code may or may not apply).

An inaccurate product definition in a contract for a computer-based patient record system or a product definition that is not sufficiently detailed can result in delivery of a system that does not function properly as a patient record system or in a contract that does not require the vendor to deliver a system that has certain important features or the capability to perform crucial patient record functions.

It is common for system vendors to "puff" the capabilities of their products in their marketing materials and in their proposals to health care providers or to promise software or features that are still on the vendor's drawing board. Although some contracting strategies help to minimize puffery and vaporware, no currently available mechanism provides complete protection against such practices.

In addition, software licenses may present problems. If a software license is not sufficiently broad in scope or duration, a provider can find itself paying unexpected additional license fees to maintain its system. An insufficiently broad license could also leave a provider without rights to use software that is crucial to the functioning of its patient record system.

Access to the source code for software is essential to a health care provider's ability to support and maintain patient record application software. Therefore, the provider should attempt to obtain a copy of the source code, either as part of the initial license grant or in the event that the vendor breaches its support obligations or decides to discontinue supporting the software. Bankruptcy, particularly among small vendors, may make it more difficult, or even impossible, to obtain the source code from a software escrow or in the event the vendor discontinues its software support.

If software licensed or sold in connection with a patient record system infringes the intellectual property rights of another, the consequences to the provider that acquires the system can be severe—both in terms of liability and loss of the right to use the software. Therefore, vendors should be required to warrant that they own the software being licensed or have the right to sublicense it. In addition, the vendor should agree to indemnify the provider and hold it harmless against claims by third parties asserting that the software or the provider's use of the software, or both, infringes on their proprietary rights.

Of course, none of the legal remedies available to a health care provider for a patient record system vendor's breach of contract is as desirable as the vendor's performance of the acquisition agreement. Therefore, it is important to structure payment schedules and conditions to payment in such a way as to give the vendor incentives to perform the agreement.

The vendor should be required to warrant that the record system will meet key performance standards, such as system response time, capacity, and batch-processing capabilities. The use of such software mechanisms as viruses and keylocks to enforce a purchaser's obligation to pay for software is becoming increasingly common, particularly among smaller vendors. Because the law in this area is still unclear, the provider should insist on a warranty in the acquisition agreement that the software does not and will never contain such mechanisms. The provider should also obtain indemnification for resulting losses and damage if such mechanisms are ever used in the acquired software. Contractual limitations on the vendor's liability should be avoided because they may leave a provider without recourse to the vendor when a patient record system fails to function or malfunctions. Such limitations on liability include limitation on the dollar amount of damages, exclusion of liability for consequential damages, limitation of liability for a provider's use of a system, and limitation of remedies to special remedies (e.g., termination and refund rights).

For health care providers who use shared computing services for a patient record system, patient record confidentiality is of special concern because the computing service receives copies of (and possibly maintains the originals of) the provider's patient records. The contract should require the computing services vendor to maintain strict confidentiality and to give the provider all necessary access to patient records (including but not limited to returning the data in usable form to the provider when the relationship ends). In addition, the contract should require the vendor to cooperate with the provider to prevent discovery of data by third-party litigants when disclosure is not legally required.

OVERCOMING LEGAL BARRIERS TO COMPUTER-BASED PATIENT RECORDS AND RECORD SYSTEMS

Adoption of Uniform National Licensure Standards and Health Information Laws

Uniform national standards should be developed for patient records maintained by health care institutions. Such requirements could be enacted at the federal or state level; however, given that regulation of health care providers falls within classic state police powers, development of uniform state licensure standards for patient records would be preferable to enactment of federal requirements. The chief disadvantage of achieving national uniformity through uniform state laws is that enacting such laws may be a lengthy process or may never actually occur. In addition, state legislatures may adopt amendments to the uniform act before enacting it as legislation. Nevertheless, the success of other uniform state legislation (e.g., the Uniform Commercial Code) suggests that such legislation could be developed and enacted by all 50 states. If enacted, these uniform state licensure standards for medical records should be applicable to all institutional health care providers that are required to maintain patient records.

The problems arising from obsolete and ambiguous state licensure standards for medical records could be resolved by the development and enactment of uniform state licensure standards expressly applicable to computer-based records and record systems. These standards should be clearly stated with respect to automated creation, authentication, storage, and retention of patient records, but should not be so detailed as to inhibit future improvements in technology.

In order to protect the confidentiality of health records and to provide patients rights of access to their health records and the right to include corrections to information in health records, all states should adopt uniform health care information legislation such as the Uniform Health-Care Information Act. Adoption of such legislation should make patients more willing to disclose sensitive information related to their health status and to have that information recorded in their health records.

If such uniform legislation were in place, health care providers presumably would have less concern about unauthorized disclosure and misuse of sensitive patient information and should, therefore, be less hesitant to record sensitive patient information in a computer-based patient record. If legislation were passed obligating third parties to whom patient information is disclosed to protect the confidentiality of such information, abuse of patient information and invasions of patient privacy should decrease. In addition, if health care information laws were uniform across all states, the applicable law would be clear and uniform, regardless of whether patient data were stored in the same state in which patients were located.

Adoption by all states of uniform health care information legislation such as the Uniform Health-Care Information Act would provide predictable access by patients to their health records and would ensure their being able to correct (or at least protest) inaccuracies contained in such records.

Overcoming Special Legal Risks Related to Computer-based Patient Records

Most of the special legal risks connected with computer-based patient records that are enumerated in this paper can best be reduced by development of new and better computer technology, including software specifically designed to reduce these risks. The greatest legal risk from computer-based patient record keeping comes from unauthorized access to record systems and from computer viruses and other sabotage, particularly in cases in which computer networks are used and there is telephone access to the patient information system. Research efforts should be directed toward developing affordable computer security technology that can adequately protect patient records without severely reducing system user friendliness.

The following would also help to reduce the potential legal risks associated with computer-based systems:

• Technological advances that make computer-based record systems more reliable and development of enhanced backup capabilities would decrease the legal risks, as well as the risks to patients, that arise when computer-based records become inaccessible.

• Development of new storage media or technology that increases and ensures the long-term durability of records stored on optical disks and other currently available media would decrease the risks arising from the uncertain or inadequate durability of current computer-based patient records.

• More reliable equipment and software for computer-based patient record systems and better mechanisms for checking and correcting human input errors would help to reduce the risks that arise from inaccurate computer-based patient records.

CONCLUSION

The promise offered by fully computer-based patient records for improving the quality of patient care and advancing medical knowledge through research is enormous. Therefore, concerted efforts should be made to overcome legal and technological barriers that stand in the way of full development of computer-based records and record systems.

In the future, with increasing use and development of artificial intelligence systems, computer-based patient records may be expected to become interactive, providing diagnostic assistance and even treatment recommendations. An interactive patient record promises improved quality of care, but the interaction of such "smart" systems with computer-based patient records will also raise a host of legal and policy issues that are beyond the scope of this paper. Among them will be allocation of responsibility (and liability) for errors in the artificial intelligence system, whether caused by faulty hardware, faulty software, or error in the system's medical rules. The more advanced such systems become, the more questions they will generate about the practice of medicine and whether nonphysicians can use these systems to diagnose and treat patients without physician involvement. In addition, systems that can diagnose or treat patients without intervening professional involvement may be classified and regulated as medical devices under food and drug laws. Finally, these "smart" systems can be expected to lead to a redefinition of the physician's role, as they begin to perform functions that formerly only a physician could perform.

Index

C